Supervision in Human Communication Disorders

Supervision in Human Communication Disorders

PERSPECTIVES ON A PROCESS

Edited by

Martha B. Crago, M.Sc.
McGill University
Montreal, Quebec

Marisue Pickering, Ed.D.
University of Maine
Orono, Maine

A College-Hill Publication
Little, Brown and Company
Boston/Toronto/San Diego

College-Hill Press
A Division of
Little, Brown and Company (Inc.)
34 Beacon Street
Boston, Massachusetts 02108

Library of Congress Cataloging in Publication Date
Main entry under title:

Supervision in human communication disorders.

"A College-Hill publication."
Includes indexes.
1. Speech therapy — Study and teaching — Supervision.
2. Audiology — Study and teaching — Supervision. I. Crago,
Martha B., 1945-   . II. Pickering, Marisue,
1937-   . III. Ling, Daniel. [DNLM: 1. Administrative
Personnel. 2 Communicative Disorders — therapy. 3. Personnel Management — methods. WM 475 S959]
RC428.S87 1987   616.85'5'007   87–3757

ISBN 0–316–15907–7

Printed in the United States of America

To Nancy Chan, supervisor for the School of Human Communication Disorders, McGill University, whose commitment to change and development in her students, as well as in herself, has been an inspiration to me.

— **Martha Crago**

To Albert T. Murphy, Boston University, who introduced me to bodies of thought I did not know existed, who first offered me the opportunity to supervise, and who continues to serve as a model of a clinician, educator, and scholar.

and

to Phyllis Goldberg Loewenstein, my first supervisor in graduate school, who has shared with me her insights and sensitivities about human interaction since the beginning of our long and rich friendship.

__ **Marisue Pickering**

Contents

Foreword

For a profession in which the majority of members are engaged in the delivery of clinical services, speech–language pathology and audiology has been magnificently adroit at avoiding coming to grips with the complexities of the processes — both clinical and supervisory — through which those services are delivered. Of the multitudes of publications that have come from our members in the 50 years since our first journal was published, relatively few have dealt directly with the clinical process, fewer still with the supervisory process. In fact, until the early 1970s only an occasional tip of the hat was given to the important activity of supervision. Since then the number of publications on the supervisory process has increased considerably, but it is still only a minuscule portion of the total output of our profession. This book makes a major contribution to rectifying that neglect.

Supervision is the process through which academic learning is applied to the clinical world. It is through generations of supervisors that clinical skills have been passed along to clinicians whose clients we assume will benefit from those skills. As a profession we have constantly increased our requirements for *quantity* of supervision; we have not, until recently, been very concerned about its *quality*. We have assumed, as attested to by the professional standards of our organization, that anyone who is a clinician is also a supervisor. Probably there have always been those who did not believe that. Fortunately, many of them are now speaking out about how the needs of supervisors are different from the needs of clinicians.

This book does that by presenting some of the major issues related to the supervisory process. The first set is what I think of as professional/political issues — questions of status, qualifications, standards, and training. The difference between supervision in audiology and in speech–language pathology also is discussed, which is important because most of the supervisory literature has not focused on supervision of students who are in training to become audiologists. The second set of issues has to do with research on the supervisory process — we have a great need for answers to many questions. The third set involves the dynamics of the interpersonal interaction between supervisor and supervisee — what happens where the "action" is?

The people who have written this book have long been involved in the supervisory process — as supervisors, as teachers of other supervisors, as researchers, as writers, as presenters at conventions and workshops. They did not begin thinking about supervision the day before yesterday — their cumulative experience with the process is impressive and they have gone directly to the heart of many of the needs of supervisors.

The time is right for this book. Interest in supervision has been growing in recent years. The American Speech–Language–Hearing Association has moved forward in adopting a set of tasks and competencies for supervisors. Many supervisors are striving to learn more about the work they are doing.

It is, therefore, a great pleasure to write the first few words of introduction to a book that addresses so many of the currently important topics about the supervisory process in speech–language pathology and audiology.

A statement in the first chapter suggests that the development of supervision in Human Communication Disorders is analogous to stages of human development. The author proposes that we are approaching a period of adolescence. This is an apt analogy for the present time, and one which we should remember as we struggle toward a better understanding of our roles as supervisors.

A young child said to me, "*Every tomorrow* I go to the swimming pool." May "every tomorrow" bring us, as supervisors, closer to a mature adulthood.

Jean Anderson, Ed.D.
Professor, Department of
Speech and Hearing Sciences
Indiana University

Preface

T his book is a collection of perspectives on the process of supervision. The chapters, written by professionals in the field of Human Communication Disorders, present ideas that go beyond the current textualized focus of supervisory practice. The book is divided into three sections: Professional Perspectives, Research Perspectives, and Interpersonal Perspectives.

The first section focuses on professional dimensions of supervision. Chapter 1 documents the history and the present state of supervision and speculates on its future possibilities as a developing speciality for speech–language pathologists and audiologists. In Chapter 2, the focus is on audiology supervision. The author not only explicates the unique nature of this type of supervision, but also addresses specific facets of its practice. This first section concludes with Chapter 3, which concerns career development issues that relate to supervisors in Human Communication Disorders. In particular, patterns of career development as explained in the Human Resource Management literature are presented and applied to the situation of the master's degree supervisor.

The second section examines research and the nature of inquiry. Chapter 4 views the research on supervision from a critical perspective. It identifies the content areas of research, the methodologies used, and the problematic dimensions of supervisory research. Chapter 5 contextualizes the humanistic, person-focused nature of the supervisory process and discusses approaches to knowing: the traditional, natural science approach as well as the interpretive-phenomenological approach. The impact of these approaches on the clinical and supervisory encounter is described.

Section three presents perspectives on the interpersonal nature of the supervisory process. Chapter 6 discusses self-exploration as a central concept in speech–language pathology supervision. A specific training program for the development of self-exploration in both students and supervisors is described. Chapter 7 identifies interpersonal dynamics that may occur in the supervisory process. These dynamics are illustrated in a series of scenarios of interactions between supervisees and supervisors. The final chapter of the book, Chapter 8, presents themes from two major bodies of literature: humanistic-existential thought and interpersonal communication. These themes are used to elucidate the nature of interpersonal communication in the supervisory process.

During the last several years, the field of Human Communication Disorders has shown an increased commitment to supervisory preparation and supervisory issues. For example, the American Speech–Language–Hearing Association (ASHA) Committee on Supervision has generated substantive discussion on supervisory training and coursework. Furthermore, the number of presentations on supervision at the annual ASHA convention and the number of refereed articles on supervision in professional journals has increased markedly. To respond to the need for supervisory preparation, American and Canadian universities are teaching courses specifically in supervision as part of their curricular offerings in Human Communication Disorders. It is now recognized that being a good clinician does not automatically mean being a good supervisor.

Although there is a growing need for academic information on supervision, there is a paucity of books on the subject. In presenting a series of perspectives on supervision, this book provides a starting point for those with a beginning interest in supervision, as well as in-depth reading for those who are more experienced supervisors. All those individuals involved in some way with the clinical teaching dimension of Human Communication Disorders should find aspects of this book relevant. This includes students, supervisors, and academic teaching faculty. In addition, sections of this book should be of particular interest to those professionals engaged in work-setting supervision of other professionals. Finally, clinical teachers in related areas of specialization may find specific chapters applicable to their work.

Supervision — clinical teaching — plays a unique role in the preparation of practitioners in Human Communication Disorders. The perspectives presented in this volume are intended to speak to selected aspects of the overall supervisory process.

Acknowledgments

As editors, we want to thank our university colleagues for their help and encouragement. For their contributions to the training program described in Chapter 6, Judy Fish and Louise Getty of the Université de Montréal deserve particular mention. Other individuals, in our departments as well as at other universities in both Canada and the United States, were kind enough to read draft copies of manuscripts, share ideas, and provide support. A heartfelt word of appreciation must be given to our secretaries, Nancy Smith of the University of Maine and Liz Morales of McGill University, for their skills and patience, particularly when we asked them to put a manuscript through the word processor "one more time." Our families, especially our spouses, Barry Crago and John Pickering, provided the kind of support and reinforcement that goes beyond what one has a right to expect — even of families — and we thank them with great affection. We also would like to acknowledge our students — the "supervisees" — and our supervising colleagues for their questions and insights over the years. Without the continual queries of such individuals, this book would be unnecessary. Finally, we want to thank our authors for their responsiveness and cooperation. A special thanks to Daniel Ling, our sponsoring editor, for his insight and guidance, and to Kirti K. Charan for the encouragement to produce this book.

Our authors also have acknowledgements:

Sandra Ulrich would like to acknowledge F. Thomas Ulrich and Thomas G. Giolas for dependable advice, encouragement, and support.

Judy Rassi would like to thank Laura Ann Wilber for her computer consultancy.

Elizabeth Gavett would like to express her thanks to Nicholas Bankson, who has served as a mentor during her years as a clinical supervisor. She is appreciative of his support, guidance, and friendship. She also would like to thank Joan Hargrave for her editorial assistance and her never-ending words of encouragement.

Vicki McCready, David Shapiro, and Kathleen Kennedy would like to acknowledge Connie Prater for her word-processing expertise, MacGregor S. Frank for editorial assistance, the staff and faculty at the University of North Carolina-Greensboro, especially Rex Prater, Cindy King, and Josephine Macon, for their support, and the staff and faculty of Western Carolina University for their support.

Contributors

Martha B. Crago, M.Sc.
School of Human
  Communications Disorders
McGill University
Montreal, Quebec

Donald G. Doehring, Ph.D.
School of Human
  Communication Disorders
McGill University
Montreal, Quebec

Elizabeth Gavett, M.A.
Department of
  Communication Disorders
Boston University
Boston, Massachusetts

Kathleen Kennedy, Ph.D.
Communication Disorders
  Program
Department of Speech
Washington University
Pullman, Washington

Vickie McCready, M.A.
Department of
  Communication and Theatre
Division of Communication
  Disorders

University of North
  Carolina at Greensboro
Greensboro, North Carolina

Marisue Pickering, Ed.D.
Department of Speech
  Communication
University of Maine
Orono, Maine

Judith A. Rassi, M.A.
Department of Communication
  Sciences and Disorders
Program in Audiology and
  Hearing Impairment
Northwestern University
Evanston, Illinois

David Shapiro, Ph.D.
Department of Human Services
Program in Communication
  Disorders
Western Carolina University
Cullowhee, North Carolina

Sandra Reimer Ulrich, M.A.
Department of Communication
  Sciences
The University of Connecticut
Storrs, Connecticut

PART I:

Professional Perspectives

CHAPTER 1

A Developing Specialty

Sandra Reimer Ulrich

S upervision has emerged as an area of specialized study and practice within the profession of audiology and speech–language pathology. In this chapter, both the past and present states of supervision in Human Communication Disorders will be discussed and its future will be speculated upon.

PAST AND PRESENT

Even though the area of supervision is a part of the earliest history of the American Speech-Language-Hearing Association (ASHA), the specialty as it is known today has been represented in the literature of the profession only since 1964 (Villareal) and emerged as a singular concept in 1978 with the publication of a Special Report from the ASHA Committee on Supervision (ASHA, 1978). In that report, a definition of the term *supervisor* appeared, and a distinction was made between two major sets of supervisory tasks: clinical teaching tasks and program management tasks. The Committee emphasized that although program management tasks may be a part of a supervisor's job duties, it is the tasks of clinical teaching that are central to the supervisory process. Clinical teaching was defined as "the interaction between supervisor/supervisee in any setting which furthers the development of clinical skills of students or practicing clinicians as related to changes in client behavior (ASHA, 1978, p. 479). The same report defined the supervisory process as "the interaction that takes place between the supervisor and the clinician and may be related to the behavior of the clinician or the client or to the program in which the supervisor and clinician are employed" (p. 479). These definitions refined the concept of supervision in Human Communication Disorders and provided direction for the development of the specialty as it exists today.

The following two sections of this chapter describe the development of knowledge and organizational structures in Human Communication Disorders supervision.

Development of Knowledge

In Human Communication Disorders supervision, there are four areas of consideration that have been of particular interest in understanding the development of knowledge:

1. Impact of practice
2. Emergence of academic offerings
3. Development of standards
4. Building of a data base

Impact of Practice on Development

Supervision clearly has been influenced by the location of where it is practiced and by its traditional population of student supervisees. The predominance of two practice settings appears to be a major factor in its development.

Supervisory practices within school practicum settings were a motivation for early attention to both the objectives and methodology of supervision (ASHA, 1978; Anderson, 1970, 1972, 1974, 1980). For speech-language pathology students, practicum in school settings often provided the major clinical experience supervised by individuals who were not employees of the college or university training program. School personnel, students, and the training programs all perceived a need for better information on expectations, responsibilities, and procedures for the supervised experience. These needs led to attempts to describe and standardize the supervisory process and to consideration of supervision's goals and objectives.

As both the number and size of university graduate education programs increased, additional numbers of persons were employed specifically to provide clinical supervision. The location of large numbers of supervisors in college or university program settings has strongly influenced definitions of supervision and supervisory roles. Daily responsibility for the development of speech–language pathologists and audiologists led to increased investigation of efficient and effective supervisory methodologies for use with students. Furthermore, concerns for recognition within both the profession and academe contributed heavily to supervision's issues and organizational structures.

The specialty's emphasis on student supervision within public schools and university programs may have precluded giving needed attention to other settings and populations. Supportive personnel, working professionals, persons in the Clinical Fellowship Year, and supervisors themselves also need supervision and, therefore, are of concern in the preparation of supervisors and the study of the supervisory process (Ulrich, 1985).

Emergence of Academic Offerings

The number of academic offerings in Human Communication Disorders supervision has been limited. Pickering (1985a) reported that 35 different universities are known to teach regular courses in supervision, although it can be assumed that there are additional programs with at least sporadic offerings. Only one university, however, is known to offer a formal educational program specific to supervision. The Indiana University program, in existence since 1972, prepares persons at the doctoral level to supervise, conduct research in the supervisory process, teach others to be supervisors, and teach others to conduct research on the supervisory process (Anderson, 1981, 1985).

Supervisors repeatedly express a strong desire for training in supervision (Anderson, 1972, 1974; Schubert & Aitchison, 1975; Stace & Drexler, 1969). Furthermore, a succession of ASHA committees concerned with supervision has urged establishment of additional academic offerings in the supervisory process (ASHA, 1972, 1978, 1985b).

Development of Standards

Standards, guidelines, and position statements are instrumental in the emergence of a profession. Supervision is in the early stages of being influenced by official documents that regulate or give direction to its practice. A major milestone was reached in 1985 with the Position Statement on "Clinical Supervision in Speech–Language Pathology and Audiology" (ASHA, 1985b). This document delineates supervision as an area of special interest, knowledge, and skills within the profession. A review follows of the steps in its development and its major content.

When the ASHA Committee on Supervision was established in 1974, two of the six items in its charge referred specifically to recommending standards and guidelines for supervisors and supervision. Responsibility for all standards later passed to the Council on Professional Standards in Speech–Language Pathology and Audiology, which developed suggested competencies for effective clinical supervision through a subcommittee. Concurrently, the ASHA Committee on Supervision, working from its original charge, developed recommendations for minimal qualifications of supervisors. The products of the two committees were published in a joint report, "Minimum qualifications for supervisors and suggested competencies for effective clinical supervision" (ASHA, 1982).

Commentary from the ASHA membership on the suggested competencies was largely positive. Responses to the mimimal qualifications, however, expressed grave concerns about the profession's ability to implement the recommendations (e.g., availability of special training, credentialing mechanisms).

With the dissolution of the Standards Council subcommittee, responsibility for the competencies passed to the Committee on Supervision. The competencies subsequently became a major focus of the 1985 Position Statement, "Clinical Supervision in Speech–Language Pathology and Audiology" (ASHA, 1985b), which eliminated the recommendations of specific educational requirements for supervisors but suggested ways in which the competencies for effective supervision could be achieved and implemented.

Traditionally, the profession has attempted to ensure the quality of its practitioners through entry-level standards. By mandating certain academic and practicum requirements, it has assumed that competence is achieved. Thus, the Position Statement's emphasis on achieving competence in specific tasks through demonstration of particular skills was a marked departure from the usual approach.

The 1985 Position Statement indicates two other milestones in the continually evolving concept of the specialty:

1. The reflection of supervision as a process with both analytical and interpersonal dimensions
2. Expression of the tasks and competencies of supervision as a responsibility shared by supervisors and supervisees.

Major contributions of the Position Statement are listed in Appendix A. The 13 tasks of supervision, identified in the Statement, are shown in Appendix B. In addition to the tasks, the Statement provides a set of competencies for each task and outlines ways in which they may be achieved.

Building a Data Base

Supervision has experienced difficulty in defining a theoretical structure and developing a basic body of knowledge that would form a nucleus of understanding for its practitioners. One reason for the difficulty has been the profession's reluctance to recognize supervision as an area of expertise worthy of specialized study. Until approximately 10 years ago, publication policies of ASHA discouraged consideration of research in the supervisory process for publication in the *Journal of Speech and Hearing Disorders* and the *Journal of Speech and Hearing Research,* which are commonly viewed as the research journals of the association.

Another reason for supervision's relatively meager representation in the literature of the profession is that the quality of supervisory research has not always been able to meet the high standards of the profession's scholarly journals and convention technical sessions. Culatta (1984) explored reasons why manuscripts on any subject failed to pass the scrutiny of editorial review for *Asha.* Although he specifically cautioned against attempts to overgeneralize findings, the seven categories that emerged from his review may assist in understanding rejections from a broad range of journals.

A related reason for the relatively small number of carefully conducted studies has been a paucity of individuals with the necessary skills to conduct such research. As noted earlier, only one doctoral level program prepares persons specifically for leadership in the area of supervision. Doctoral dissertations in the supervisory process are rare from other universities, although they have been done (e.g., Caracciolo, 1977; Engnoth, 1974; Oratio, 1978; Pickering, 1979). Because it is doctoral studies that are assumed to be the preparation for research activity, the small number of persons who are prepared at that level *and* interested in pursuing supervisory research has hampered the research effort. Nevertheless, master's degree level professionals could learn research skills, a point made by Laney (1982) in her discussion of research in the public schools. Kennedy (1985) suggested that the tendency to view master's level supervisors as incapable of research activities may be "person-based or position-based" (p. 34).

Butler (1976) addressed the problem from another perspective when she noted the difficulties of quantifying supervision's complex matrix. Shapiro (1985) approached the issue from yet another direction when he noted wide variations in theories and techniques of inquiry, and "a relative paucity in the methodology and machinery for testing (them)" (p. 93). Nevertheless, when Butler (1980) later reviewed research efforts between 1960 and 1980, she noted increasingly sophisticated attempts to resolve issues and concluded, "The art of supervision is evolving into a science" (p. 13).

Any discussion on building a data base must look at where dissemination of research actually occurs. Certainly supervision articles do exist in all four journals of the American Speech–Language-Hearing Association. In addition, *The Clinical Supervisor* is a major resource for information about the supervisory process in general. Persons from Human Communication Disorders are frequent contributors to this journal and also serve on its editorial board.

Papers and other documents about supervision can be shared through use of ERIC, a nationwide network to collect and make available educational documents and papers. Pickering (1985b) provided information on using ERIC for both dissemination and acquisition of manuscripts or other materials. *SUPERvision,* the quarterly publication of the Council of University Supervisors of Practicum in Speech–Language Pathology and Audiology (CUSPSPA), is particularly suited to dissemination of research findings and other information about supervision.

In addition to print resources, supervisors have used conventions and conferences to share information. In 1983, ASHA's annual convention was enhanced as a vehicle for dissemination by creation of a special subcommittee to the Program Committee. This committee, known as Professional Affairs II, reviews proposals in the area of education and training issues and specifically includes clinical supervision in its purview. Drawing on Culatta's (1984) work, Pickering (1984) discussed the review process for convention proposals and outlined reasons for rejection. The large number of presentations about supervision at recent conventions, however, suggests that these gatherings provide a major forum for dissemination of information about the specialty.

In the 1960s and 1970s, a series of conferences and workshops concerning supervision (Anderson & Kirtley, 1966; Anderson, 1970; Conture, 1973; Turton, 1973) led to later focus on supervision as a specialty area. A national conference at Indiana University in 1980 provided a forum for supervisors from throughout North America to discuss important current issues in supervision. CUSPSPA assumed responsibility to schedule a second national conference on supervision in 1987. Regional, provincial, state, and local conferences provide additional opportunities for dissemination.

Development of Organizational Structures

In this section, the organizational structure of supervision in the United States and Canada as it has existed until now will be described. The organizational structure of supervision remains largely informal. Nevertheless, some structures are in place through the Council of University Supervisors of Practicum in Speech–Language Pathology and Audiology (CUSPSPA), ASHA, the Canadian Association of Speech–Language Pathologists and Audiologists (CASLPA), and other groups.

Council of University Supervisors of Practicum in Speech–Language Pathology and Audiology (CUSPSPA)

The primary opportunity for supervisors to identify with a formal structure is afforded by CUSPSPA. In 1970, persons with shared concerns for supervision of school practicum formed a group known as the College and University Supervisors of School Practicum. Interests for supervision of practicum in varied settings soon emerged, and, in 1974, this group became the Council of University Supervisors of Practicum in Speech–Language Pathology and Audiology.

Membership is open to speech–language pathologists and audiologists who have earned at least a master's degree or its equivalent in communication disorders or, at an associate level, to students actively pursuing a degree in the discipline. Until recently, membership was restricted to persons who had earned the Certificate of Clinical Competence (CCC) from ASHA, but constitutional changes now allow associate membership status, with no voting privileges, to individuals without a CCC who meet other requirements for membership. The change was motivated by the group's desire to permit participation by persons active in supervision in Canada, where the CCC is not a credential for practice. Nevertheless, the Council's continuing requirement that voting members hold the CCC demonstrates its interactive relationship with standards promulgated by ASHA.

CUSPSPA shows annual membership rolls that average approximately 250 members. It has members in most states and several provinces, an annual meeting during the ASHA convention, and a quarterly publication (*SUPERvision*) that carries articles and news about supervision, as well as book reviews and summaries of convention papers. Its educational and research network (SUPERNET) coordinates supervisory research and assists in organizing regional and state supervisory associations and programs. CUSPSPA also has an informal working relationship with the ASHA Committee on

Supervision, and a CUSPSPA member is appointed annually to serve as a liaison to the ASHA Committee. A joint project was undertaken by the two groups in 1986.

CUSPSPA serves as a resource for information about the supervisory process and as an advocacy group for the practice of supervision. The personal contacts established through CUSPSPA have served a networking function for supervisors throughout the United States and Canada. In addition to its programs and publications, CUSPSPA has assisted individuals in recognizing, applying, and further investigating the body of knowledge and skills that constitute the practice of supervision.

As its title implies, the concerns and activities of CUSPSPA concentrate on supervision of students. Membership requirements do not exclude participation by persons whose supervisory responsibilities are with other populations of supervisees (e.g., professional clincians), but the purposes of the group emphasize student supervision (CUSPSPA, 1982).

Even though CUSPSPA is the national and international organization for supervisors, its membership is relatively small. No definitive information exists concerning the number of people who supervise students, although Pickering (1985a) suggested that as many as 5000 persons may be engaged in supervision related to college and university programs. If this figure is accurate, with a membership of only 250, CUSPSPA represents just five percent of this group.

American Speech–Language–Hearing Association

Recognition for the role of supervision in preparing persons as speech–language pathologists and audiologists is found in early membership requirements of the American Speech–Language–Hearing Association, but it was not until the 1960s that concerns for supervisory roles and skills were expressed in the literature of the association (Halfond, 1964; Van Riper, 1965; Ward & Webster, 1965a, 1965b). The interactive relationship of ASHA and supervision during the 20 years between 1964 and 1984 is shown in Appendix A.

COMMITTEE ON SUPERVISION IN SPEECH–LANGUAGE PATHOLOGY AND AUDIOLOGY. With establishment in 1974 of the Committee on Supervision in Speech Pathology and Audiology (later changed to Speech–Language Pathology and Audiology), ASHA demonstrated its commitment to the area of supervision and recognition of supervision's role in a variety of settings. The Committee's 1978 Special Report identified nine priority needs in supervision (see Appendix A) and recommended ways in which those needs might be met. Its 1985 Position Statement (ASHA, 1985b) was a direct result of recommendations in the 1978 Special Report. The significance of the Position Statement has been noted earlier and is re-emphasized here.

The Position Statement outlines three ways in which the skills and competencies for effective clinical supervision may be obtained:

1. Specific curricular offerings from graduate programs
2. Continuing educational experiences specific to the supervisory process
3. Research-directed activities that provide insight into the supervisory process

The Statement calls for establishment of additional opportunities for preparation of supervisors "both within and outside graduate education programs" (p. 60) and affirms the need for "systematic study and investigation of the supervisory process" (p. 60). The activities of the Committee on Supervision continue, in part, to focus on the preparation of supervisors.

The Committee provides a vital link with the profession for the area of supervision and for supervisors.

OTHER ASHA COMMITTEES. Further evidence of ASHA's commitment to supervision is found in the large number of boards, committees, and task forces with responsibilities or concerns in the area of supervision. Groups such as the Clinical Certification Board and the Committee on Supportive Personnel have responsibilities related directly to supervision. Other committees are charged with tasks for which supervision is an implied concern, for example, committees that deal with special programs or settings in which supervision occurs (e.g., Committee on Quality Assurance, Task Force on Home Care).

Canadian Association of Speech–Language Pathologists and Audiologists (CASLPA)

Within CASLPA, interest in supervision is reflected in national, provincial, and regional activities. Persons with particular concerns about supervision met during the 1982 annual meeting of CASLPA to form the Committee of University Coordinators of Supervision in Speech–Language Pathology and Audiology. Although the Committee exists as a related professional group, rather than an official body of CASLPA, its major activity occurs as a part of association meetings. In addition, CASLPA's publication, *Human Communication Canada,* is the major vehicle in Canada for publication of articles concerned with supervision, and its conventions provide a forum for papers and other presentations in the specialty area (e.g., Crago, Getty & Fish, 1983; Crago & Godden, 1986; Ellis, 1980; Hatten, 1986; Heaton, 1983). With fewer than 3000 practicing speech–language pathologists and audiologists in Canada, CASLPA has developed along lines that are somewhat different from ASHA. Nevertheless, the commitment to supervision is one of its strong characteristics.

Other Groups

In 1985, the Council of Graduate Programs in Communication Sciences and Disorders devoted a major portion of its annual conference to the area of clinical supervision. The following three resolutions concerning supervision and the role of supervisors in graduate education were adopted (Bernthal, 1985):

1. Recognition of supervision as a teaching function; establishment of a committee to study terminology relative to titles of clinical supervisory personnel, procedures for the evaluation of supervisory personnel, and career advancement for such personnel
2. Direction to member programs to initiate avenues for personal and professional development
3. Direction to member programs to expand opportunities for participation of supervisory personnel in program decision-making

A national joint committee, composed of representatives from the Council, CUSPSPA, and the ASHA Committee on Supervision, was established to meet the intent of the first action.

In the United States, state and regional groups interested in supervision have formed and often are affiliated with state professional associations or with CUSPSPA. For example, formal or informal associations are known to exist in the states of Illinois, Indiana, Ohio, and Virginia, and, in recent years, the New England states have joined for an annual conference about supervision. Recent correspondence with a group of supervisors in the college and university education programs of New Zealand to the ASHA Committee on Supervision suggests that concerns for supervision and the supervisory process are not restricted to North America.

Summary: Past and Present

The first two sections of this chapter demonstrate increasingly sophisticated delineation of major issues in Human Communication Disorders supervision, with positive achievements in some areas. There is good evidence that supervision is equipped with strategies and organizational structures for continued acquisition of the knowledge and skills that constitute its evolving concept and practice.

THE FUTURE

In this section, attention will be drawn to a set of issues that must be considered as supervision moves into the future. Some of these issues are already being addressed by the organizational structures of the specialty. Others await further refinement before strategies of resolution can be developed. All provide evidence, however, that the concept and practices of supervision are not static in nature and will continue to evolve.

Preparation of Supervisors

The need to prepare supervisors is no longer a question for the future. As previously mentioned, the ASHA Committee on Supervision considers this a priority, and its Position Statement outlined three avenues of supervisory preparation. The major goal of preparation is the mastery of the "Competencies for Effective Clinical Supervision," which constitute the major portion of the Position Statement.

Smith and colleagues (1985) presented models for preparation in the supervisory process. Included were a doctoral level emphasis, examples of postgraduate coursework and practicum, a continuing education model, an audiology emphasis, and models that include preservice coursework as an introduction to the supervisory process. Major issues in the preparation of supervisors include accessibility, funding, qualified teachers, employment opportunities for supervisors, and employer recognition of the specialized study. Anderson (1981) has outlined some obstacles to the creation of supervisory training programs in university settings that are also applicable to other settings.

Issues within the profession will also affect the preparation of supervisors. For example, any major changes in the certification process or structure could alter the demand for supervisors, the tasks and skills of supervision, or the form and content of supervisor preparation. Other issues, such as specialty certification, outcome of the standards validation study, and doctoral-level entry to the profession would have similar impact.

The evolution of supervision to date has been influenced remarkably by attention to specific concerns at concentrated points in time. Using only recent history as an example, the 1970s could be described as the decade of interaction analysis systems, followed in the 1980s by a focus on the complexities of the supervisory conference. Even now, however, a shift is being observed, with attention directed more and more to preparation of supervisors. It has been noted repeatedly in this chapter and elsewhere that much of the demand for training comes from supervisors themselves. As the specialty continues to develop, it must come to grips with the issues inherent in the preparation of its practitioners.

Concerns of ASHA

The future of supervision undoubtedly will continue to be affected by events within the profession of speech–language pathology and audiology. The following areas of concern are related to issues being addressed by ASHA: standards validation, certification and licensure, and quality assurance.

Standards Validation

Perhaps no issue can be expected to have as great an impact on supervision as that which will come from the standards validation study currently underway (ASHA, 1984). An external firm works with ASHA on this project to independently validate certification requirements.

The resulting product will be a validated list of job tasks with the associated knowledge, skills, and abilities necessary for their execution. This list then will be linked to the academic and clinical practicum requirements of the CCC, the national examinations in speech–language pathology and audiology, and the Clinical Fellowship Year (CFY).

If estimates are correct for numbers of persons who devote some portion of their time to supervision, there is little doubt that supervisory tasks should be identified through standards validation study, with subsequent attention to this responsibility in the standards program of the profession. Some persons who engage in supervision, however, do so with a limited concept of the supervisory process and little knowledge of its skills. Thus, participants in the standards validation sample could fail to recognize the supervisory activity in their daily routines, might categorize supervision as an administrative task, and could describe the supervisory process in only a cursory manner. Rassi (1985) acknowledged that to the occasional beholder, supervision may appear to be a "simplistic task requiring little effort or knowledge beyond the clinical routine" (p. 27). The possibility that such a viewpoint could be reflected in the sample for the standards validation study needs to be recognized. A finding of this nature would be a setback of extraordinary proportions in the development of supervision.

Certification and Licensure

Issues of certification and licensure that are separate from the matter of standards validation continue to be studied by ASHA. They too will shape the development of supervision. What credential will determine supervisory competence to its consumers (i.e., employers and supervisees)? Some states already have regulations for special credentialing of school supervisors or coordinators. It is highly likely, however, that the requirements for supervisors of speech, language, and hearing services in these settings have been determined by persons without special knowledge of the supervisory process, and it is almost certain that these decision-makers are unfamiliar with the specific skills of supervision in Human Communication Disorders. Establishing independent registries of persons deemed to have particular expertise in the specialty area of supervision might be a viable option for clinical supervisors.

Quality Assurance

Quality assurance is another area that will affect supervision. It is an area, however, that offers opportunities for the specialty of supervision to influence and assist the profession. A basic premise of the ASHA standards program, as well as those of other agencies, is that regulations can help to ensure quality of individual professionals, of educational and training programs, and of service delivery. The ultimate goal is protection of the consumer.

ASHA established a Committee on Quality Assurance in 1975 and charged it with the responsibility of developing a system of accountability. Currently, work is underway for development of a performance appraisal system that would address the competence and performance of individual practitioners, as well as for the development of guidelines for standards of care (ASHA, 1985a).

Traditionally, supervisors have filled a quality assurance role in the delivery of services by analyzing and evaluating both the performance of the supervisee and the quality of care being provided. Flower (1984), for example, notes that supervision "may well be the oldest, most traditional approach to quality assurance" (p. 297). Guidelines that offer criteria for their judgments should be welcomed by supervisors. It is essential, however, that persons responsible for application of the guidelines be trained in the process of analyzing, evaluating, and modifying clinical performance. In other words, these persons must be trained in clinical supervision.

Decline in Student Enrollment

Reports indicate that the number of persons applying to graduate programs in speech–language pathology and audiology is diminishing, and concerns have been raised about the quality of students preparing for the profession (Lingwall & Snope, 1982; Punch & Fein, 1984). Fewer students in educational programs would suggest a decline in the number of supervisory positions. On the other hand, if the professional quality of these students is diminished, the need for closer, more frequent, and more skillful supervision would seem apparent in educational programs and in other work settings.

The supply of future supervisors is closely related to the issue of a decline in numbers and quality of students entering the profession. Reductions in the quantitative and qualitative pool of potential supervisors would result in the need to selectively recruit supervisors and would underscore the critical need for additional resources of supervisor preparation and training.

Funding Factors

Reductions in federal funding, changes in state or provincial tax revenues, and changes in administrative priorities have been, and will continue to be, issues affecting both training programs and clinical services programs. Supervisory positions are affected in at least two ways:

1. In training programs, supervisory positions often are funded through training grants, so that as these funds are decreased or

eliminated, financial support for the supervisory position disappears. Further, as universities seek ways to reduce expenses, the positions most vulnerable to layoffs are those outside the tenure system or those faculty who have not yet achieved tenure; most clinical supervisors fall into these categories. Both the profession and the specialty need to address the question of how supervisory positions can be retained. More important, however, is the basic question of how students will be supervised if supervisory positions are eliminated. If increased supervisory responsibilities are assigned to remaining faculty, it will be necessary for them to learn and apply the knowledge and skills that constitute supervision.

2. In clinical services programs, changes in entitlement programs or their enabling legislation (e.g., Medicare, Medicaid, P.L. 94-142) as well as in reimbursement policies of commercial insurers, directly affect the very existence of these programs. Numbers of persons seeking services, as well as the extent of services that are affordable to the individual or the agency, can change rapidly with changes in funding. Numbers of supervisory positions may change, or reductions in other staff may modify the workloads and tasks assigned to supervisors. It thus becomes important for supervisors to document and advocate the contributions of supervision to both quality and efficiency of service programs.

Audiology Supervision

In Chapter 2, Rassi compares supervision in the two areas of practice and discusses the special strategies and methodologies emphasized in audiology supervision. Although she believes that much of the study in speech–language pathology supervision is not directly applicable to audiology, Rassi's thoughts, in fact, have contributed markedly to a framework for speech–language pathology supervision. The eight levels of interaction and "stations" that she outlined (1978) assist all supervisors, regardless of their area of practice, in recognizing and implementing small increments of sequential change in the supervisor–supervisee interaction. In addition, many of the techniques used in audiology supervision are applicable to speech–language pathology supervision of assessment activity, where the constraints on preplanning, supervisor intervention, client responsiveness, and postevaluation client counseling are similar. Other concerns of the audiology supervisor are frequently raised by speech–language pathology supervisors in a variety of settings. These concerns include record keeping, efficiency of service to the client, use of technical equipment, and nonconference approaches to supervisee feedback. Thus, it appears that at least some of the differences between audiology and speech–language pathology supervision may reflect variations in the relative frequency of assessment and treatment activity or may be related to the particular work environment. Audiology and speech–language pathology supervision should assist each other in resolving their common concerns.

Supervisee Populations

There is an urgent need for supervision to apply its knowledge and skills to supervisees other than students. Its principles and goals are appropriate throughout the professional careers of speech–language pathologists and audiologists, as well as in the work of paraprofessionals and volunteers. Earlier it was implied that the supervisors of these populations are less likely to identify with the specialty area, or even to recognize that information and guidance is available to assist them in carrying out their supervisory responsibilities. Heaton (1983) noted some basic differences in the type of supervision required when dealing with practicing clinicians rather than with students and mentioned some modifications of function. Nevertheless, new skills need to be developed throughout professional careers; new clients present unique challenges to the interpersonal domain of the clinical process; and new information emerges to assist clinicians in self-analyzing, self-evaluating, and self-directing, all of which are facilitated through supervisory interactions.

The 1985 Position Statement on Clinical Supervision emphasizes a colleagueship between supervisor–supervisee that is particularly relevant to varied levels of training and experience. Supervisors of experienced clinicians or paraprofessionals, however, often see their roles as administrative in nature or as a part of program management tasks. Often, the administrator or manager of a service program supervises the other staff. These people may not necessarily understand or desire the responsibility of supervision. In addition, issues similar to those mentioned for audiology supervision (e.g., time constraints, emphasis on productivity) may seem incompatible to forms of supervision developed for students. Research on supervision may appear irrelevant to supervisee populations other than students.

The concept of supervision in the future, the tasks that constitute its practice, and its strength as a specialty area will reflect the degree to which needs of multiple supervisee populations are considered and included in its membership.

Off-Campus Supervision

The use of off-campus practicum sites is highly variable from one university to another. In some programs, off-campus practicum may begin early in a student's program. In others, it is reserved largely for an externship semester. Many issues of off-campus supervision are identical to those in on-campus settings. Other specific difficulties are related to the off-campus supervisory experience.

Off-campus supervisors have limited contacts with the training program. Even though most universities maintain schedules of periodic off-campus visits or telephone contacts, the off-campus supervisor is less familiar with items such as the training program's curriculum and philosophy, examination schedules and other constraints on students' time, prior academic and clinical performance of the student, criteria for evaluating clinical skills, and the university's expectations for the practicum experience than is an on-campus counterpart.

Ehrlich and colleagues (1983) explored several issues related to the economic support of off-campus supervision, and Rassi (1985) examined some assumptions concerning field supervisors, most of which she believed to be mythical. Some of the issues related to off-campus supervision can be solved through better communication or special projects. For example, Brasseur (1985) and Casey (1985) reported on coursework and supervisory practica developed specifically for off-campus supervisors, with generally positive conclusions about the trainees' enthusiasm for the offerings and improved relationships between the training programs and their off-campus supervisors. Ulrich (1983) outlined information necessary both to and from universities, students, off-campus facilities, and off-campus supervisors for effective off-campus experiences. Moreover, in Chapter 6, Crago gives a detailed description of the preparation of off-campus supervisors.

Economic issues are not so easily resolved. Off-campus sites often face administrative pressures to increase revenues and sometimes experience their own loss of funding and staff positions. They may become unable to provide supervised experiences to students, regardless of personal commitment.

Influence of Technology

Supervision per se often is not considered a high technology practice. Its major tools in many settings continue to be paper, pencil, and tape recorder. The picture is changing rapidly. Supervision in the future can expect increasing influence from, for example, videotaping, distance learning, and computer technology.

Videotaping

Supervisors use video and audio recording for demonstration and teaching of clinical skills, as an adjunct to direct observation and data collection, as an avenue for facilitating the self-analysis and self-evaluation skills of supervisees, and as a rehearsal tool for clinical activities as diverse as history-taking and client staffings. Recent advances in video technology that have resulted in miniaturization and allow low-light filming make it possible to record in a variety of settings not previously considered in supervision (e.g., homes, small clinic rooms and offices, test suites). Further, the technology offers ways for supervisors-in-training to observe conferencing skills, to practice analysis of both clinical and supervisory interactions, and to be supervised themselves. These examples suggest that videotaping will continue to be a major tool used to enhance the supervisory process.

Distance Learning

Distance learning includes teleconferences and other packaged programs of instruction. It provides opportunities for individuals or groups in widely scattered locations to have access to experts on specific topic areas. In the teleconference format, remote sites are connected to an originating source of live instruction; special equipment allows participants to communicate with the instructor for questions, discussion, and so on. Packaged programs of instruction usually consist of an instructional manual and audio- or videotape, although they may be comprised of only written materials. An examination may be included, which is completed and returned to a central source for scoring and feedback of results to the individual. Distance learning offers exciting possibilities for supervisory preparation and a practical way to bring experts on supervision to a large number of individuals at relatively low cost.

Computers

Specific challenges and opportunities are created for supervision by the microcomputer revolution. For research, statistical programs permit treatment of data at a level of sophistication previously considered by only a few supervisors. Similarly, the ability of computers to store, sort, and analyze relationships among large amounts of separate information allows supervision to study the complex nature of its process in innovative ways. Furthermore, clinical and supervisory record-keeping is facilitated by computers. Computer-aided instruction for both students and clients, scheduling, report generation, cost analysis, client assessment, hearing aid selection, and augmentative communication are other examples of computer applications of special interest to supervisors. The ability of computers to allow communication across long distances suggests that there may be new supervisory formats to consider, as well as possibilities for teaching clinical skills and for management of clients unable to regularly visit clinic settings. The concept of interactive computer instruction is only beginning to be explored, but the process is underway and must be considered in the future of supervision.

Networking

Supervisors frequently have turned to each other for interpersonal and emotional support and have been able to provide nurturing, reassurance, and judgment validation to each other in extraordinary ways. As the number of persons identifying with supervision increases, the specialty will need to find ways to extend networking opportunities without distancing its practitioners from its structures and without the internal struggles for power that often are a part of other groups. The ability to retain a strong *esprit de corps* is a challenge to the future of supervision.

Individual Responsibility

More than anything else, the future of supervision will depend on supervisors themselves — as a group and as individuals. Supervisors must be willing to identify and address issues and must develop and implement strategies for their resolution.

Even though supervisors argue their rights to self-direct, it sometimes appears as though they are waiting for others to provide data, define roles, and offer solutions. It is essential for *individual* supervisors to assume responsibility in their own work settings for the following:

1. Demonstrating the effects of supervision
2. Defining their roles with administrators
3. Ensuring that the hierarchical system of the work place understands and accepts the defined role and accommodates it in its policies and procedures for job security and promotions

4. Utilizing mechanisms to document the quality of their clinical and supervisory skills

To carry out these activities, supervisors will need to consult the literature and use the supervisory network. Most importantly, *individual* supervisors must understand that they contribute to the evolving concept of the specialty.

During recent years, the assertiveness of supervision in claiming its rightful place within the profession has brought long-sought recognition to the specialty. This was not accomplished solely by the efforts of individual supervisors, however. Support and assistance came from many and varied sources, for example, university administrators, colleagues in teaching and research, and professional association leaders and peers. Supervisors, as a group and as individuals, need to recognize that the bureaucracy is not an adversary and that status for the specialty is now a reality. The time has come for supervisors to identify resources to meet the challenges ahead and to learn appropriate ways to utilize these resources for shaping the future of the specialty.

Summary: Supervision in the 21st Century

In the remaining chapters of this book, perspectives on the concept and practice of supervision are described. In this chapter, the development of the specialty has been looked at, and topics that appear to be important in shaping future evolution of supervision in Human Communication Disorders have been discussed.

Earlier it was suggested that the 1985 Position Statement from the ASHA Committee on Supervision in Speech–Language Pathology and Audiology marked a new and significant level in the development of supervision. This event occurred exactly 13 years after the appointment of the professional association's first task force concerned with supervision. Analogies to the stages of human development would label this a coming of age and suggest a subsequent period of adolescence.

If this is a correct analogy, certain predictable patterns of growth may be expected. Supervision will assert its uniqueness as a specialty area. It will seek, test, discard, modify, and adapt the thinking of others and generate ideas of its own. It will move from a position of dependence on its progenitors, both within and outside the profession, to one of looking to its peer groups across disciplines to provide substantial portions of nurturing and validation. It will also mature from a largely egocentric beginning to a stage in which it contributes to others and demonstrates its competence to self-analyze and self-direct.

Supervision today is impatient with its own growth and evolution. It wishes to be free of its imposed boundaries and to have its worth be better recognized. It is still uncomfortable with itself and yet excited about the future — somewhat universal traits of adolescence. In a recent interview with *The Hartford Courant,* a marketing executive was asked, "Are you what you expected to be?" His answer was:

"The only expectation I've ever had for myself is that I be the best that I can. And that is an evolutionary process. So I'm comfortable with where I am (now), knowing that it's somewhere less than I expect of myself for the course of my life." (O'Neill, 1986, p. 6)

Supervision expects the best from itself. It expects to be somewhere else in the 21st century. Its foundations are positive. The characteristics of its adulthood will be evident by the ways it meets the challenges of today.

REFERENCES

American Speech and Hearing Association, Task Force on Supervision in the Schools. (1972). Supervision and continuing professional education. Task force report. *Language, Speech, and Hearing Services in Schools, 3*(3), 3–17.

American Speech and Hearing Association, Committee on Supervision in Speech Pathology and Audiology. (1978). Current status of supervision of speech–language pathology and audiology. Special report. *Asha, 20,* 478–486.

American Speech–Language–Hearing Association, Committee on Supervision in Speech–Language Pathology and Audiology. (1982). Minimum qualifications for supervisors and suggested competencies for effective clinical supervision. *Asha, 24,* 339–342.

American Speech–Language–Hearing Association, Ad Hoc Committee on Standards Validation. (1984). *Standards validation study.* Unpublished report. Rockville, MD.

American Speech–Language–Hearing Association. (1985a). Minutes of the Executive Board Meeting, August. Rockville, MD.

American Speech–Language–Hearing Association, Committee on Supervision in Speech–Language Pathology and Audiology. (1985b). Clinical supervision in speech–language pathology and audiology. A position statement. *Asha, 27*(6), 57–60.

Anderson, J. L. (Ed.). (1970). *Conference on supervision of speech and hearing programs in the schools.* Bloomington, IN: Indiana University.

Anderson, J. L. (1972). Status of supervision in speech, hearing, and language programs in the schools. *Language, Speech, and Hearing Services in the Schools, 3*(1), 12–22.

Anderson, J. L. (1974). Supervision of school speech, hearing, and language programs — an emerging role. *Asha, 16,* 7–10.

Anderson, J. L. (Ed.). (1980). *Proceedings. Conference on Training in the Supervisory Process in Speech–Language Pathology and Audiology.* Bloomington, IN: Indiana University.

Anderson, J. L. (1981). Training of supervisors in speech–language pathology and audiology. *Asha, 23,* 77–82.

Anderson, J. L. (1985, November). Doctoral level emphasis. In *Preparation and training models for the supervisory process.* Short course presented at the meeting of the American Speech–Language–Hearing Association, Washington, DC.

Anderson, J. L. & Kirtley, D. (Eds.). (1966). *Institute on supervision of speech and hearing programs in the public schools.* Indianapolis, IN: Department of Public Instruction.

Bernthal, J. E. (Ed.). (1985). Proceedings on the Sixth Annual Conference on Graduate Education. Lincoln, NE: University of Nebraska, Council of Graduate Programs in Communication Sciences and Disorders.

Brasseur, J. A. (1985, November). External/internal practicum. In *Preparation and training models for the supervisory process.* Short course presented at the meeting of the American Speech–Language–Hearing Association, Washington, DC.

Butler, K. (1976, November). *The supervision of clinicians: The three C's . . . competition, complaints and competencies.* Paper presented at the meeting of the American Speech–Language–Hearing Association, Houston, TX.

Butler, K. (1980). Supervision issues in speech–language pathology and audiology: A personal and professional perspective. In J. L. Anderson (Ed.), *Proceedings. Conference on Training in the Supervisory Process in Speech–Language Pathology and Audiology* (pp. 7–26). Bloomington, IN: Indiana University.

Caracciolo, G. L. (1977). Perceptions by speech pathology student clinicians and supervisors of interpersonal conditions and professional growth during the supervisory conference. (Doctoral dissertation, Teachers College, Columbia University, 1976). *Dissertation Abstracts International, 37,* 4411B.

Casey, P. L. (1985, November). Course and practicum at graduate level. In *Preparation and training models for the supervisory process.* Short course presented at the meeting of the American Speech–Language–Hearing Association, Washington, DC.

Conture, G. (1973). *Special study institute: Management and supervision of programs for speech and hearing handicapped.* Unpublished manuscript, Syracuse University, Syracuse, NY.

Council of University Supervisors of Practicum in Speech–Language Pathology and Audiology. (1982). Constitution. *SUPERvision, 6*(1), 8–10.

Crago, M., Getty, L. & Fish, J. (1983, May). *A supervisors' workshop.* Presentation at the annual conference of the Canadian Speech and Hearing Association, Montreal.

Crago, M. & Godden, A. (1986, May). *Evaluation and dissonance in supervision: A supervisor-supervisee exchange.* Presentation at the annual conference of the Canadian Association of Speech-Language Pathologists and Audiologists, Winnipeg.

Culatta, R. (1984). Why articles don't get published in Asha. *Asha, 26*(3), 25-27.

Ehrlich, C. H., Merten, K., Sweetman, R. H. & Arnold, C. (1983). Training issues: Graduate student externship. *Asha, 25*(12), 25-28.

Ellis, E. (1980, May). A perspective of issues affecting speech and hearing. In *Supervision in speech-language pathology and audiology in Canadian employment settings.* Presentation at the annual conference of the Canadian Speech and Hearing Association, Winnipeg.

Engnoth, G. (1974). A comparison of three approaches to supervision of speech clinicians in training (Doctoral disseratation, University of Kansas, 1973). *Dissertation Abstracts International, 39,* 6261B.

Flower, R. M. (1984). *Delivery of speech-language pathology and audiology services.* Baltimore, MD: Williams & Wilkins.

Halfond, M. (1964). Clinical supervision — stepchild in training. *Asha, 6,* 441-444.

Hatten, J. T. (1986, May). *Strategies of supervision in diverse settings.* Presentation at the annual conference of the Canadian Association of Speech-Language Pathologists and Audiologists, Winnipeg.

Heaton, E. (1983). Minimum qualifications for supervisors. *Human Communications Canada, 6,* 380-382.

Kennedy, K. (1985). Hidden dynamics related to the supervisory role. In J. E. Bernthal (Ed.), *Proceedings of the Sixth Annual Conference on Graduate Education* (pp. 33-39). Lincoln, NE: University of Nebraska, Council of Graduate Programs in Communication Sciences and Disorders.

Laney, M. D. (1982). Research and evaluation in the public schools. *Language, Speech, and Hearing Services in Schools, 13,* 53-60.

Lingwall, J. B. & Snope, T. L. (1982). *Today's students in speech-language pathology and audiology: Some quantitative and qualitative changes.* Rockville, MD: American Speech-Language-Hearing Association.

O'Neill, A. (1986). Are you what you expected? Interview in *Northeast Magazine.* Hartford, CT: *The Hartford Courant,* February 16.

Oratio, A. R. (1978). Multivariate relationships between clinician-client demography and discrete therapeutic behaviors, as perceived by clinical supervisors. (Doctoral dissertation, Bowling Green State University, 1979). *Dissertation Abstracts International, 38,* 4173-B.

Pickering, M. (1979). Interpersonal communication in speech-language pathology clinical practicum: A descriptive, humanistic perspective (Doctoral dissertation, Boston University, 1979). *Dissertation Abstracts International, 40,* 2140-41B. (University Microfilm No. 79-23, 892).

Pickering, M. (1984). Why some ASHA convention proposals didn't get accepted by the professional affairs II subcommittee. *SUPERvision, 8*(2), 12–15.

Pickering, M. (1985a). Clinical supervision in a university setting: Overview of the topic. In J. E. Bernthal (Ed.), *Proceedings of the Sixth Annual Conference on Graduate Education* (pp. 15–19). Lincoln, NE: University of Nebraska, Council of Graduate Programs in Communication Sciences and Disorders.

Pickering, M. (1985b). Share your ASHA presentation through ERIC. *SUPERvision, 9*(3), 21–22.

Punch, J. L. & Fein, D. J. (1984). Profile of educational programs in speech-language pathology and audiology. *Asha, 26*(1), 43–48.

Rassi, J. (1978). *Supervision in audiology.* Baltimore, MD: University Park Press.

Rassi, J. (1985). Competencies, qualifications, training: Audiology. In J. E. Bernthal (Ed.), *Proceedings of the Sixth Annual Conference on Graduate Education* (pp. 26–32). Lincoln, NE: University of Nebraska, Council of Graduate Programs in Communication Sciences and Disorders.

Schubert, G. W. & Aitchison, C. J. (1975). A profile of clinical supervisors in college and university speech and hearing training programs. *Asha, 17,* 440–447.

Shapiro, D. A. (1985). Clinical supervision: A process in progress. *Journal of the National Student Speech Language Hearing Association, 13,* 89–108.

Smith, K., Anderson, J., Brasseur, J., Casey, P., Ganz, C., Laccinole, M., McCrea, E., Rassi, J. & Ulrich, S. (1985, November). *Preparation and training models for the supervisory process.* Short course presented at the meeting of the American Speech-Language-Hearing Association, Washington, DC.

Stace, A. & Drexler, A. (1969). Special training for supervisors of student clinicians: What private speech and hearing centers do and think about training their supervisors. *Asha, 11,* 318–320.

Turton, L. (Ed.). (1973). *Proceedings of a Workshop on Supervision in Speech Pathology.* Ann Arbor: University of Michigan, Institute for the Study of Mental Retardation and Related Disabilities.

Ulrich, S. R. (1983, September). *Supervision in speech-language pathology.* Workshop at Hahnemann University, Philadelphia, PA.

Ulrich, S. R. (1985, November). Continuing education model of training. In *Preparation and training models for the supervisory process.* Short course presented at the meeting of the American Speech-Language-Hearing Association, Washington, DC.

Van Riper, C. (1965). Supervision of clinical practice. *Asha, 7,* 75–77.

Villareal, J. (Ed.). (1964). *Seminar on Guidelines for Supervision of Clinical Practicum.* Washington, DC: American Speech and Hearing Association.

Ward, L. & Webster, E. (1965a). The training of clinical personnel: I. Issues in conceptualization. *Asha, 7,* 38–40.

Ward, L. & Webster, E. (1965b). The training of clinical personnel: II. A concept of clinical preparation. *Asha, 7,* 103–106.

APPENDIX A.
Chronology of ASHA/Supervision Interaction

1964: ASHA-sponsored seminars
   1. Seminar on Guidelines for Supervision of Clinical Practicum in Training Programs[1]
   2. Seminar on Guidelines for Internship Year[2]

1970: Task Force on Supervision in the Schools established; report published 1972[3]

1973: Task Force statements and recommendations incorporated into two manuals:
   1. *Program Planning, Development, Management, and Evaluation: A Manual for School Speech, Hearing, and Language Programs*[4]
   2. *Standards and Guidelines for Comprehensive Language, Speech, and Hearing Programs in the Schools*[5]

1974: Committee on Supervision in Speech Pathology and Audiology established with following charge:[6]
   1. Promote and disseminate the current information about supervision in speech pathology and audiology
   2. Promote research on the supervisory process
   3. Identify significant issues in supervision in training programs, the Clinical Fellowship Year, and in various employment settings
   4. Recommend standards and guidelines for the roles and responsibilities of supervisors in the settings listed in Item 3
   5. Develop strategies for encouraging the employment of supervisory personnel
   6. Recommend standards and guidelines for training programs in supervision

1978: Special report of Committee published; nine issues identified for priority consideration.
   1. Data to validate the supervisory process
   2. Role definition for supervisors specific to the context of the various work settings in which they work
   3. More supervisors

4. Better quality in the supervision that is currently being provided
5. Special standards for supervisors, other than the Certificate of Clinical Competence
6. Training for supervisors
7. Investigation of the status of supervisors, particularly within the academic system
8. Investigation of the ambiguities and problems that exist in the supervision of the Clinical Fellowship Year
9. Accountability systems for supervisors

1984: Position Statement accepted by Legislative Council and published 1985:[8]
1. Defines supervision as distinct area of expertise and practice
2. Outlines 13 special tasks of supervision
3. Describes competencies for each task
4. Provides suggestions on how competence may be achieved
5. Calls for additional preparation opportunities

---

[1]Villareal, J. (Ed.) (1964). *Seminar on guidelines for supervision of clinical practicum.* Washington, DC: American Speech and Hearing Association.

[2]Kleffner, F. (1964). *Seminar on guildines for the internship year.* Washington, DC: American Speech and Hearing Association.

[3]American Speech and Hearing Association, Task Force on Supervision in the Schools. (1972). Supervision and continuing professional education. Task force report. *Language, Speech, and Hearing Services in the Schools, 3*(3), 3–17.

[4]American Speech and Hearing Association. (1973). *Program planning, development, management, and evaluation: A manual for school speech, hearing, and language programs.* Rockville, MD.

[5]American Speech and Hearing Association. (1973–74). *Standards and guidelines for comprehensive language, speech, and hearing programs in the schools.* Rockville, MD.

[6]American Speech–Language–Hearing Association. (undated). *Manual of resolutions adopted by the legislative council.* Rockville, MD

[7]American Speech and Hearing Association, Committee on Supervision in Speech Pathology and Audiology. (1978). Current status of supervision of speech–language pathology and audiology. Special report. *Asha, 20,* 478–486.

[8]American Speech–Language–Hearing Association, Committee on Supervision in Speech–Language Pathology and Audiology. (1985). Clinical supervision in speech–language pathology and audiology. A position statement. *Asha, 27*(6), 57–60.

APPENDIX B.
Tasks of Supervision

1. Establishing and maintaining an effective working relationship with the supervisee
2. Assisting the supervisee in developing clinical goals and objectives
3. Assisting the supervisee in developing and refining assessment skills
4. Assisting the supervisee in developing and refining clinical managment skills
5 Demonstrating for and participating with the supervisee in the clinical process
6. Assisting the supervisee in observing and analyzing assessment and treatment sessions
7. Assisting the supervisee in the development and maintenance of clinical and supervisory records
8. Interacting with the supervisee in planning, executing, and analyzing supervisory conferences
9. Assisting the supervisee in evaluation of clinical performance
10. Assisting the supervisee in developing skills of verbal reporting, writing, and editing
11. Sharing information regarding ethical, legal, regulatory, and reimbursement aspects of professional practice
12. Modeling and facilitating professional conduct
13. Demonstrating research skills in the clinical or supervisory process

American Speech-Language-Hearing Association, Committee on Supervision in Speech-Language Pathology and Audiology. (1985). Clinical supervision in speech-language pathology and audiology. A position statement. *Asha, 27*(6), 57-60.

CHAPTER 2

The Uniqueness of Audiology Supervision

Judith A. Rassi

The uniqueness of audiology supervision derives from the uniqueness of clinical audiology itself. Like many other clinical areas, audiology may be viewed as having the traditional diagnosis–evaluation component and the traditional therapy–(re)habilitation–treatment component. Nevertheless, depending on individual job specifications according to work setting, the relative emphasis of these two components may not be equal. Most audiologists are primarily involved in evaluation and hearing aid work, along with audiological counseling and preliminary or basic aural rehabilitation. There is usually no involvement or only secondary involvement in therapy-based aural rehabilitation programs (Schow, 1986). Thus, audiology supervision is directed more toward evaluation activity than toward therapy activity.

Supervisory approach is determined by what constitutes a clinical activity (e.g., a sequence of diagnostic inquiry, assessment, deduction, and advice-giving) rather than by the nature of the disorder itself. In audiology, supervision may be patterned after models in a number of fields. If evaluation is primary and therapy is secondary, applicable models may be found in the health care professions, in medicine, industry, and business management. Conversely, if therapy is the major clinical emphasis and evaluation plays a minor role, audiology supervisory approaches are modeled appropriately after those in teacher education, psychology, social work, and speech–language pathology.

In the field of Human Communication Disorders,[1] the supervision literature, convention presentations, and research studies are based almost exclusively on speech–language pathology. Thus, given the prevalence of therapy in speech–language pathology work and the prevalence of evaluation in audiology work, much of this supervision information is not directly applicable to audiology. Audiologists can look at supervision data from the field of Human Communication Disorders for certain kinds of information, but they must draw from other fields for relevant principles, guidelines, and procedures.

A comparative analysis of audiology supervision with speech–language pathology supervision reveals basic characteristics — some different, some similar — that influence the respective supervisory approaches. The differences include:

- Number and variety of clients involved
- Number of return visits pairing a client and a supervisee
- Number of supervisees assigned per supervisor per clinical session
- Allotted time for completion of clinical and supervisory tasks
- Physical environment as it relates to the placement of supervisor, supervisee, and client
- Physical closeness of supervision along with the associated need for error detection
- Observation and intervention moves by a supervisor
- Use of technical equipment and devices
- Frequency and format of supervisory conferences
- Practicability of direct versus indirect supervisory styles

The basic similarities between audiology supervision and speech–language pathology supervision are fewer in number and more general in nature. The most obvious of these similarities is the

---

[1]The author recognizes and supports the concept of a single disciplinary base focusing on human communication and its disorders (the field) and that of a single profession providing delivery of services to individuals with communication disorders, as both are proposed in the American Speech-Language-Hearing Association's (ASHA) position statement on a single profession and its credentialing (ASHA, 1982) and delineated by Moll (1983) at the National Conference on Undergraduate, Graduate, and Continuing Education. Nevertheless, Moll (1983) acknowledges further that there are specifically defined areas of practice — namely, speech–language pathology and audiology. It is these separate areas of practice that pertain to this chapter's ideas on speech–language pathology supervision versus audiology supervision.

involvement in the clinical–supervisory process of a client with a communication disorder. It is interesting that this property linking the two clinical areas has also been viewed as their mutual base for supervisory approaches. As indicated earlier, however, the nature of the clinical disorder is not necessarily a supervision factor. Another more binding similarity between the two areas is their mutual goal of developing a supervisee's clinical skills. Finally, there is the similarity, the bond, that ties together not only speech–language pathology supervision and audiology supervision but all spheres of supervision: the broad range of personal interactions between supervisor and supervisee. This theme prevails in supervision presentations and transcends the uniqueness of any single field.

FEATURES OF AUDIOLOGY SUPERVISION

Audiology supervision has distinguishable features that have come to characterize its essence. Even though audiology supervision is a process, it has definitive and constant characteristics, which are discussed below.

Competency-Based Instruction

Competency-based instruction has been viewed as a skill-building task (Rassi, 1978) that incorporates accountability for meeting established objectives (Anderson, 1974). When the supervisory process in audiology is examined according to these propositions, competency-based instruction emerges as a key characteristic (Rassi, 1978). It is especially suitable for audiology supervision because the nature of clinical audiology permits a ready dissection into competency parts. A delineation of identifiable, teachable competencies has been illustrated previously in the form of four audiology skill–competency scales for testing, writing, interpersonal, and decision-making areas (Rassi, 1978). Specific audiology competencies appear in the appendices at the end of this chapter.

Another example of competency delineation is found in the ASHA's comprehensive listing of supervision tasks and their corresponding competencies for effective clinical supervision (ASHA, 1985). Although these particular tasks and competencies were written expressly for supervisors, most of them can be converted directly into clinical competencies, that is, the competencies to be taught to supervisees by supervisors.

Competency-Based Goal-Setting and Evaluation

Competency-based instruction is the logical basis for competency-based goal-setting and competency-based evaluation. Goal-setting can be accomplished through joint planning and discussion by the supervisor and supervisee at or near the beginning of a practicum assignment. With preparatory knowledge of the supervisee's educational background and clinical practicum experience and of the specific clinical competencies to be attained, the supervisor and supervisee can set appropriate goals. This goal–setting process is facilitated further by predetermining the expected mimimal achievement levels for each of the competencies. As shown in excerpts from the sample form Expected (Minimal) Achievement Levels for Students in Clinical Practicum and Competency-Specific Evaluation Criteria (Appendix A), expectation levels can be designed to correspond with supervisee developmental stages in a clinical practicum sequence.

Competency-based evaluation can occur at any time that a supervisor and supervisee might wish to examine a supervisee's progress toward goal attainment. Either one or both individuals may elect to have ongoing review or to conduct evaluations at typical midterm and end-of-term junctures. Evaluation items in a competency-based framework can simply and directly refer back to their respective goals. This is shown in excerpts from the form Evaluation of Student in Clinical Practicum (Appendix B). At any time during the evaluation process, this system allows comparison of current performance status to a previous expectation or intention.

In educational programs in which a supervisee's clinical performance is graded, competency-based grading is the logical result of competency-based goal-setting, instruction, and evaluation. Grading criteria can be based on a supervisee's actual attainment of expected minimal achievement levels. This is indicated in the sample document Grading System for Audiology Practicum (Appendix C). Such a system connects prepracticum goals to postpracticum evaluation. Moreover, a competency-based approach to clinical grading may be viewed as being more equitable to those being graded and more justifiable by those doing the grading than other approaches. This was found to be the prevailing response in a survey of supervisor and student reactions to goal-oriented, competency-specific evaluation and grading (Rassi, 1979).

Competency-based goal-setting and evaluation also enhance the possibility of self-evaluation by the supervisee. For example, self-evaluation can be facilitated by the delineation of specific competencies. Supervisee self-evaluation may be assisted further by the systematic self-monitoring that can come about in pursuing a goal. Finally, there is the likelihood of increased self-evaluation during supervisory feedback exchanges when supervisees reflect on their reasoning processes.

Skill Development

A competency-based view of audiology supervision allows a concentration on skill development. In his analysis of supervision in counseling psychology, Hart (1982) observed that a skill development model of supervision emphasizes a teacher–student relationship between the supervisor and supervisee. Purtilo (1984) indicated that skills, along with theoretical knowledge and attitudes, constitute the kinds of learning that take place in a health professional's education. Her steps of skill acquisition, as listed here, are particularly applicable to audiology supervision (Purtilo, 1984, pp. 5–6):

The student:
1. Acquires background knowledge related to the skill,
2. Experiences the skill applied to himself or herself,
3. Applies the skill to a normal classmate,
4. Observes a professional person using the skill,
5. Assists the professional person using it,
6. Is closely supervised in the first attempts to use it alone,
7. Satisfactorily uses it in a variety of situations without direct supervision, and
8. Is tested for mastery of skill.

Although the first of these steps takes place in the classroom and the second and third take place in laboratory settings, thereby leaving the remaining steps for clinical practicum, it is not uncommon for audiology supervisors to find themselves also responsible for certain components of the initial steps.

Orderly skill development requires careful planning and strategic maneuvering on the part of the audiology supervisor because of the ever changing complexity of the clinical cases (Rassi, 1978). In a typical clinical facility, difficult cases are intermixed with those requiring less clinical skill, regardless of the supervisee's developmental stage at any given time. Skill development in audiology practicum supervisees is also limited by the (sub)variety of cases available for them to evaluate or manage. A further complication is the difficulty many student clinicians have in adapting skills to a wide range of case types. As a consequence, expectations for skill development may not be met (Ehrlich, Merten, Sweetman & Arnold, 1983).

Skill development related to clinical evaluation seems especially appropriate in the realm of audiology supervision because of the many step-by-step operational procedures and methodical decision-making processes used. Of equal importance, however, is the development of interpersonal skills in the supervisee. The history-taking, the audiological counseling, and the client management and rehabilitation aspects of clinical audiology, when considered together, require a substantial investment of supervisory time and effort. Although these particular activities have their own skill-building agenda, it is their interpersonal dimension that audiology supervisors need to emphasize through role-modeling as well as through instructional techniques. Interpersonal skill development in supervisees likely requires as much, or perhaps more, systematic supervisory planning as does the development of other clinical skills. It cannot be assumed that student clinicians have adequately developed interpersonal skills for clinical work (Klevans, Volz & Friedman, 1981).

Supervision Strategies

Knowing the goals to be attained and the skills to be developed by a supervisee, the audiology supervisor can devise applicable supervision strategies. Strategies may incorporate either instructional (Rassi, 1978) or collegial (Cogan, 1973) approaches or an approach that focuses on skill development as well as personal growth in the supervisee. Whatever specific audiology supervision strategies are used, however, the following factors should be taken into account.

Principles of Learning

In their work at the Center for Educational Development at the University of Illinois Medical Center in Chicago, Foley and Smilansky (1980) found that certain generally accepted learning principles have consistent application to instruction in the health professions. Such principles have particular relevance in this context:

• The student should be provided opportunities to be an active rather than a passive learner.

• The student should be provided opportunities for understanding the logic underlying teaching activities.

• The student should have the opportunity to learn through a variety of educational resources (e.g., small-group discussions promote more problem solving but are less appropriate for skills development than structured practice sessions).

• The student should be provided with models which serve as criteria for the expected performance.

• Until the expected level of competence is attained, students should have adequate opportunities to practice using the knowledge and skills they have learned and receive feedback on their performance.

• Students should be provided with opportunities to examine ways of adapting learned knowledge and skills based upon the characteristics of a given situation.

• Overall, students should have learning experiences which are positive and satisfying rather than negative and frustrating (Foley & Smilansky, 1980, pp. 94–97).

Although these principles appear to be accepted and used in the typical audiology supervisor's armamentarium of clinical teaching techniques, this author has observed during individual supervision consultations and group supervision seminars that application is less than consistent. On becoming aware of their importance in clinical learning, however, the supervisors involved have incorporated such principles effectively into regular supervisory planning as well as in practicum design.

Levels of Supervision and Supervision Stations

Supervision in audiology occurs at different levels of interaction and at different supervisory stations (Rassi, 1978). As indicated in the following list, there are eight identifiable levels of interaction, ranging from the first and most direct where the supervisor models clinical activities for the supervisee, to the eighth level, which finds the supervisor's participation confined to monitoring and consultation.

1. Detailed explanation, with accompanying demonstration, of every action from beginning to end of test session.

2. General explanation, with some accompanying demonstration, of every action from beginning to end of test session.

3. Suggestions or corrections while student is performing task(s) under close supervision.

4. Prestructuring of task(s) beforehand, with no explanation while student is performing task(s).

5. Instruction of student on what task is to be performed and its underlying rationale, but no explanation of how to do it before, during, or after task performance.

6. Review beforehand with student of task(s) to be performed with student making all decisions; accompanying suggestions only when necessary.

7. Review of task(s) with student only after he or she has completed them.

8. Student makes all decisions, performs all tasks alone, with supervisory monitoring and suggestions only when deemed necessary (Rassi, 1978, p. 15).

Supervision stations refer to the physical placement of the supervisor in relation to the supervisee and the client during the clinical-supervisory process. As with the levels described, Rassi (1978) identified 8 corresponding supervision stations, with the first being the closest — supervisor seated in "test chair" — and the eighth level fostering supervisee independence by placing the supervisor outside the clinic rooms, sometimes observing, sometimes not. The intermediate stations find the supervisor participating, observing, or listening at various locations within the audiology control room and test room as well as outside the test suite where clinical activity may or may not be observable.

The Use of Questions

Asking questions of students and supervisees has been a time-honored teaching tool of classroom instructors and clinical supervisors. The way in which questions are phrased and the purposes behind them need to be analyzed and understood by the questioner-instructor. Foley and Smilansky (1980) reported that questions in the clinical practicum setting can be used effectively to promote clinical problem-solving. The following points from their work stand out as being important for the clinical audiology supervisor:

• Ask predominantly open-ended questions rather than those requiring recall.

• When appropriate, probe for additional data, reasoning, possible actions.

• Ask hypothetical, speculative "what if" questions.

• Give students adequate time to think about and answer questions without interrupting with another question or with the answer.

• Encourage students to answer their own questions or those asked by others.

• Sequence questions in logical order such as: history, findings, management, follow-up; or What would you do? Why? What does it mean? What if?

• Use appropriate phrasing, that is, ask clear, concise questions rather than long, ambiguous ones that combine a number of issues; avoid repetitive questions (Foley & Smilansky, 1980, pp. 58–60).

It has been this author's observation, by means of supervision practicum, consultation, and seminar discussion, that such educational precepts were not consistently or even consciously followed by the audiology supervisors involved. Since applying newly learned techniques of question-asking, however, these same persons have noted that clinical decision-making and problem-solving by supervisees is indeed fostered this way.

Error Detection

Audiology supervisors may spend much of their observation time scrutinizing audiological records for accuracy of test results and watching supervisees operate test equipment. Although the supervisor can and should be flexible in allowing individual differences to be present in such supervisee-performed tasks, there are many omissions, substitutions, and other kinds of errors to detect, correct, and discuss. Error detection requires detailed attentiveness and a knowledge of common audiology errors.

Principles of Clinical Teaching

Examination of an audiology supervision model such as that proposed by Rassi (1978) reveals that many of the instructional tasks performed by an audiology supervisor have common elements. Thus, whether instructing a supervisee about pure-tone threshold determination or hearing aid selection, the supervisor proceeds from preview through procedural and rationale explanations to review. At specific intervals, the supervisor is expected to demonstrate techniques, ask questions, and check performance for all tasks. These recurring elements create a pattern that is enhanced by the use of specific clinical teaching principles. The following principles have been found to be directly applicable:

- General-to-specific, or categories-to-details, questions are meaningful and memorable.
- Explanation of the rationale for each action, operation, or procedure facilitates understanding.
- Informational question-asking during instruction is helpful in determining the supervisee's level of understanding.
- Concepts, when presented in a logical, skill-building order, are most clearly understood and retained in memory.
- Preview, explanation, and review of salient points are elucidative.

- Gestures and pointing, especially when working with equipment, give appropriate focus to explanations and demonstrations.

During laboratory instruction associated with an introductory supervision course taught by this author, the demonstration of these principles through role-playing has provided further evidence of their applicability in audiology supervision.

PROFESSIONAL FACTORS INFLUENCING AUDIOLOGY SUPERVISION

The nature of the professional practice of audiology influences the methods of audiology supervision. There are factors intrinsic to audiology that require particular supervisory consideration. Six such factors and their effects on supervision are identified in this section.

Technical Operations

Because of the complexity of contemporary test equipment and test procedures, of hearing aids and assistive listening devices, and of earmolds and ear impression techniques, close supervision is essential. In addition to the previously mentioned task of error detection being important, so is the need for step-by-step clinical teaching, joint problem-solving, and client safety. Also, during the manipulation of equipment and the selection of test moves, a supervisee's thinking and reasoning processes need to be probed and monitored. This must be done at the time of actual decision-making, not later.

Observation and Intervention

Because of the need for close observation, the audiology supervisor is situated physically close to the supervisee or the client. The observation that results is clearly different from nonparticipatory observation, in which the supervisor may be isolated by a one-way window and a one-way sound system. A need for immediate intervention on the part of the audiology supervisor is often also indicated. These unique close observation and immediate intervention requirements affect the dynamics among client, supervisor, and supervisee as well as the supervisory experiences involving memory, attribution and judgment matters.

Audiological Counseling

Because of the need for immediate counseling at the end of an audiological session, there is little opportunity to plan counseling strategies for each case. Thus, meeting both client and supervisee needs becomes problematic for the supervisor.

Experience suggests that audiological counseling, along with areas such as history-taking and instruction-giving, receive less supervisory attention than other competency areas. This poses a consequential supervision problem for audiology: of Hart's (1982) three common developmental stages of supervision (skill development, personal growth, and integration), interpersonal skill development may be de-emphasized and the latter two stages may be overlooked. It is ironic that because audiological client counseling is often provided within a single-visit session this clinical task is viewed by some persons as having secondary, rather than primary, importance. Such a distorted impression can misdirect the well-intentioned supervising clinician and misinform the unknowing supervisee. Appropriate supervisory emphasis on the interpersonal aspects of audiological endeavors, including client counseling, is therefore especially important to the well-rounded preparation of preprofessional audiology supervisees. The importance of practicum counseling experience has been underscored in a survey of communication disorders programs accredited by the ASHA Educational Standards Board (McCarthy, Culpepper & Lucks, 1986).

Writing

In audiology, recordkeeping and reporting requirements vary greatly — from the detailed accounts common in educational settings to the concise entries found in medical settings. In addition, the audiological reports issued in medical settings often need to be written and disseminated within minutes after the evaluation has been completed; thereby requiring immediate supervisory attention. In such situations, it may become expedient to exclude the supervisee from this clinical activity. Given the importance of teaching principles of clinical report-writing to supervisees (Sanders, Middleton, Puett & Pannbacker, 1985–1986), the audiology supervisor must frequently devise special strategies for involving supervisees. Such strategies might include:

• Brief discussion and collaboration by the supervisor and supervisee, with the actual writing done by the supervisor

• Dictation of report content by the supervisor, along with rationale explanation, as the supervisee responds and writes the report
• Immediate writing of the actual report by the supervisor, followed by later supervisor–supervisee discussion as time permits.
• Subsequent homework writing of a "practice" report by the supervisee on the basis of preparatory discussion and case records.

Time Management

It is difficult for both the audiology supervisor and supervisee to find enough time for supervisory planning, instruction, and evaluation. The following factors influence this dilemma.

Work Setting

Depending on the work setting, the results of an audiological evaluation may need to be summarized almost instantly. Such is the case in most medical settings. The corollary to immediately expected results is that audiological evaluation of clients will be fast paced and efficient. The speed of evaluation often demands considerable teaching-learning compromise on the part of the supervisor and supervisee.

Hearing aid dispensaries also place unusual time demands on clinician-supervisors. Because walk-in clients must be handled between regularly scheduled appointments, timely closure must be reached on most clinical activities. The audiology supervisor's proficiency in clinical-versus-supervision time management becomes especially important.

Although it has frequently been assumed that university clinics are devoted primarily to education and secondarily to service, this is not necessarily true. Even though students' clinical education is viewed as being important, client service may often take precedence over student participation because of the time factor. For the supervising clinician, there may be no choice about intervening for the sake of quickening the test pace. Rapid audiological evaluations may result in keeping referral services, whereas slow audiological evaluations may result in losing them.

Clinical Population

In audiological evaluation, clinical population factors such as age and responsiveness have an effect on attention span and cooperation by the client. These factors can significantly alter the amount of available clinical time when successful conditioning and valid responses to test stimuli are critically dependent on a clinician's timing, pacing, and interpretational skills. Special supervisory intervention is frequently necessary to guide supervisees through problems posed by particular populations.

Feedback

Providing ongoing, nonconference feedback to supervisees is routine for the auditory supervisor. This is in contrast to the observation–conference approach associated with speech–language pathology supervision. As a result, there are few planned conferences; these usually occur at the time of midterm and end-of-term evaluations. Thus, supervisory conferences in audiology practicum are usually evaluative in nature, whereas the unscheduled ongoing feedback may be either evaluative or nonevaluative.

Nonevaluative feedback occurs not only in discussions between the supervisor and supervisee but also in supervisory role-modeling activities where the supervisor participates in the clinical session or interacts with the client and the client's family. Because role-modeling feedback, whether evaluative or nonevaluative, is not always identified by the supervisor as actual feedback, supervisees may misconstrue the feedback intention or overlook an evaluative message (Rassi, 1983a).

The promptness of the informal feedback that has come to characterize much of audiology supervision is apparently advantageous in that immediate feedback is considered to be more productive than delayed feedback (Crago, 1983; Hart, 1982). Audiology supervisors involved in supervision study have supported this premise (Rassi, 1980).

CONCERNS ABOUT AUDIOLOGY SUPERVISION

If audiology supervision, because of and in spite of its uniqueness, is ever going to attain status as a specialty area, it must address three major areas of concern.

Research and Dissemination Needs

As stated at the beginning of this chapter, speech–language pathology provides the basis for most of the literature, convention presentations, and research on supervision in Human Communication Disorders. This situation has been the cause of frustration among audiology supervisors who seek, but often do not find, directly applicable information from sources within the field. As a probable consequence of their unsatisfied informational needs, audiology supervisors attend supervision presentations and join supervision interest groups in disproportionately low numbers. Furthermore, they rarely give supervision presentations, conduct supervision research, or write supervision articles, thus perpetuating their own dilemma. Until more supervising audiologists become involved directly in information-producing and information-disseminating activities, audiology supervision will remain undeveloped as a viable area of study (Rassi, 1983b).

Appropriate supervisory process analysis and meaningful comparison of experiences and procedures with those in other areas of practice are needed to establish an original data base. Moreover, the supervision offerings by speech–language pathologists should not be ignored. Regardless of the source, many supervision presentations do contain some potentially usable or adaptable information. Audiology supervisors must recognize that certain basic elements of the supervisory process are universal, even though the areas of practice and the supervision models may differ (Rassi, 1983b).

There are several research avenues to be pursued in audiology supervision. Nonconference approaches to the study of supervisor–supervisee interactions are needed. It cannot be assumed that the many reported findings from conference analyses are applicable to the unplanned, ongoing, and situation-focused exchanges between supervisor and supervisee in audiology supervision. Another suggested research direction is the systematic examination of teaching methods for equipment operation, procedural moves, and attendant clinical decision-making. Data showing how these supervision tasks interface with other clinical education components in the laboratory and classroom settings should also be obtained. Perhaps the least obvious, but most important, direction of pursuit should be simply to increase understanding of audiology supervision, not only by the supervisors and supervisees who engage in it but also by speech–language pathology supervisors and by nonsupervisors in the field. Recognition, identification, definition, and description can serve to enhance appreciation of the process by both participants and observers.

The Changing Clinical Scene

The impact of increasingly sophisticated technology on clinical audiology and on the clinical supervision of audiology students has been remarkable and consequential. Moreover, the adoption of hearing aid dispensing as a routine activity in most clinical facilities and the corresponding need for involving practicum students in business aspects of clinical practice have significantly altered audiology clinical and supervisory processes. These compelling forces create challenges for supervising clinicians who not only must learn new and sometimes complicated clinical tasks but also must teach this information to supervisees from an assumed experiential perspective.

Proficient administration and accurate interpretation are crucial for the procedures that have been added over the years to the audiology armamentarium, for example, acoustic immittance testing, electronystagmography, measurement of auditory evoked potentials, and electroacoustic measurement of hearing aid performance. Earmold impressions are now made routinely by audiologists, as are earmold modifications, hearing aid adjustments, and minor hearing aid repairs. The focus of hearing aid selection procedures has shifted gradually from extensive, aid-by-aid, client-reported and test-score comparisons to formula-based techniques. Software programs have been developed to facilitate decision-making in the selection of hearing aids, which, not incidentally, have increased in variety and versatility. Audiometers have functions and options previously unknown, and aural rehabilitation strategies now incorporate many technological advances previously unavailable. It is evident that these dramatic advances in clinical audiology require extraordinary skill on the part of the audiology supervisor. At the same time, such developments provide another explanation as to why the continuing education efforts of audiologists are infrequently devoted to the topic of supervision.

The ever changing technology, the growing business emphasis, and the current expansion of audiology in medical and private-practice settings appear to be affecting clinical and supervisory practices in another, more subtle way. Detailed audiological counseling, as has been suggested, may be abridged in order to accommodate these and other factors, or the emphasis of audiological counseling may be shifted in a substantive or philosophical way. Notwithstanding these apparent changes in many practicum environments, preprofessional students cannot afford to miss the opportunity to develop counseling skills. Adjustments in supervision must continue to account for all of a supervisee's learning needs, not just those that serve special interests or coincide with a current development.

The Future of the University Audiology Clinic

The audiology marketplace has changed noticeably in recent years. With the increasing number of audiologists in physicians' offices, hospitals, and private-practice enterprises, the competition for clients has emerged as a critical factor in the administration of university audiology clinics. Moreover, although universities may continue to enjoy the advantages of time-honored respect and professorial resources, their clinical operations typically are not geared to offer the kind of fast, flexible, and often-abbreviated service demanded by referral sources and the consumer public. Student supervision appears to be the major reason for this difference because it necessarily takes clinical time, hence decreases the likelihood of optimal efficiency and flexibility. In addition, the loss of alternate sources of financial support and the placement of appropriate value on clinical services has led to the reduction of long-standing fee differences between university and nonuniversity services. With this change, another possible reason for choosing the university clinic has been eliminated.

The upshot of these developments is clear: If university audiology clinics are to remain viable, they must offer new services unavailable elsewhere and must market services vigorously. Given the inability of many university systems to maintain clinics that are self-supporting, these remedial measures may actually determine survival.

This difficult situation has several implications for audiology supervision. Because of its competency-based, teacher–learner paradigm, the supervisory process in audiology seems best served by pairing one supervisor with one supervisee in a particular clinical session at a given point in time. This one-to-one ratio of supervisors to supervisees has become highly desirable and, indeed, the expected arrangement in most audiology practica. Nevertheless, it imposes an enormous expense on a university education program — an expense that is becoming increasingly unaffordable in many places. With a view toward survival, university clinics must seek to develop new supervisory approaches that continue to offer practicum students the best possible learning experiences. Yet these approaches must be innovative and flexible so as not to further tax the supervision work force. Although the computerization of clinical teaching seems to be part of the answer to this dilemma, the interpersonal aspects of clinical practicum must not be neglected or sacrificed.

An alternative, which appeals to some persons in the field, but not to others (Rees & Snope, 1983), to using university (audiology) clinics for basic practicum education lies in off-campus facilities. Currently, many of these sites accept clinical students for externship assignments, which typically follow or coincide with more elementary practicum work in university clinics. A ready willingness of nonuniversity clinicians to assume added responsibility for the beginning phases of practicum should not necessarily be expected, however. Some persons in off-campus facilities who now offer externship arrangements have reported that student supervision is time-consuming and costly (Ehrlich et al., 1983). A survey of supervisors, which addressed this particular issue, revealed almost equivalent numbers of off-campus respondents agreeing and disagreeing with a statement that student supervision reduces the efficiency of a clinical service operation, hence costs both time and money (Adam, Calabrese, LeDuc, Mogil & Rassi, 1985). Even so, other considerations would be likely to enter into any decision concerning the possible transfer of basic practicum education from university clinics to off-campus sites. As indicated by Ehrlich and colleagues (1983), monetary compensation for the off-campus sites' extra work must be considered. If money becomes a factor and if universities are required to bear the compensation expense, the cost of university clinical and supervisory operations would not be solved by exporting the responsibility. Moreover, the preparedness of off-campus supervising clinicians for full-time supervisory work is problematic.

CONCLUSION

The research and dissemination needs, the changing clinical scene, and the future of the university audiology clinic form a set of concerns that will determine the course of audiology supervision. Whatever direction this course takes, it is hoped that any modifications in the present system of audiology clinical education will incorporate recognized principles of clinical teaching and learning. In addition, the unprecedented technical know-how required of audiology supervisors and supervisees should be balanced against their continuing need for counseling proficiency and refined interpersonal skills. The ultimate requisites for audiology supervision include recognition as an entity, validation of its process, and proven viability in a context of perpetual change. The research challenge is great. The need for well-educated, well-prepared audiologists and supervising audiologists is even greater.

REFERENCES

Adam, C., Calabrese, B., LeDuc, J., Mogil, S. & Rassi, J. (1985, April). *Current attitudes toward off-campus student supervision.* Panel presented at the meeting of the Illinois Council of Supervisors in Speech–Language Pathology and Audiology, Chicago, IL.

American Speech–Language–Hearing Association, Ad Hoc Committee on a Single Profession and its Credentialing. (1982). Committee report. *Asha, 24,* 407–409.

American Speech–Language–Hearing Association, Committee on Supervision in Speech–Language Pathology and Audiology. (1985). Clinical supervision in speech–language pathology and audiology. A position statement. *Asha, 27*(6), 57–60.

Anderson, J. L. (1974). Supervision of school speech, hearing, and language programs — an emerging role. *Asha, 16,* 7–10.

Cogan, M. L. (1973). *Clinical supervision.* Boston, MA: Houghton Mifflin.

Crago, M. (1983, November). *Student-supervisor interactional self-exploratory training: A description and model.* Short course presented at the meeting of the American Speech–Language–Hearing Association, Cincinnati, OH.

Ehrlich, C. H., Merten, K., Sweetman, R. H. & Arnold C. (1983). Training issues: Graduate student externship. *Asha, 25*(12), 25–28.

Foley, R. P. & Smilansky, J. (1980). *Teaching techniques: A handbook for health professionals.* New York: McGraw-Hill.

Hart, G. M. (1982). *The process of clinical supervision.* Baltimore, MD: University Park Press.

Klevans, D. R., Volz, H. B. & Friedman, R. M. (1981). A comparison of experiential and observational approaches for enhancing the interpersonal communication skills of speech–language pathology students. *Journal of Speech and Hearing Disorders, 46,* 208–213.

McCarthy, P., Culpepper, N. B. & Lucks, L. (1986). Variability in counseling experiences and training among ESB-accredited programs. *Asha, 28*(9), 49–52.

Moll, K. L. (1983). Issue II. What should be the content and objectives of graduate education in communication disorders? In N. S. Rees & T. L. Snope (Eds.), *Proceedings of the 1983 National Conference on Undergraduate, Graduate, and Continuing Education. ASHA Reports, Number 13* (pp. 25–37). Rockville, MD: American Speech–Language–Hearing Association.

Purtilo, R. B. (1984). *Health professional/patient interaction.* Philadelphia, PA: W. B. Saunders.

Rassi, J. A. (1978). *Supervision in audiology.* Baltimore, MD: University Park Press.

Rassi, J. A. (1979, November). *Goal-oriented, competency-specific evaluation for supervised audiology practicum.* Poster session presented at the meeting of the American Speech–Language–Hearing Association, Atlanta, GA.

Rassi, J. A. (1980, November). *The evolution of a training program in audiology supervision.* Miniseminar presented at the meeting of the American Speech–Language–Hearing Association, Detroit, MI.

Rassi, J. A. (1983a, November). *Evaluative and non-evaluative feedback for practicum students: A supervisors' exchange.* Miniseminar presented at the meeting of the American Speech–Language–Hearing Association, Cincinnati, OH.

Rassi, J. A. (1983b). Audiology supervision. *SUPERvision, 7*(3), 10–12.

Rees, N. S. & Snope, T. L. (1983). National conference on undergraduate, graduate, and continuing education. *Asha, 25*(9), 49–59.

Sanders, K., Middleton, G. F., Puett, V. & Pannbacker, M. (1985–1986). Report-writing: Current issues and proposed directions. *SUPERvision, 9*(4), 23–32 (Summary).

Schow, R. L. (1986). Aural rehabilitation forum: Rehabilitating the elderly hearing impaired; Audiologists as hearing aid dispensers. *Corti's Organ, 11*(1), 4–6.

APPENDIX A.

Excerpts from: *Expected (Minimal) Achievement Levels for Students in Clinical Practicum and Competency-Specific Evaluation Criteria*

This guide is to be used in conjunction with the form "Evaluation of Student in Clinical Practicum" in which the 1,2,3,4,5,X ranking system is used. Items appear in the same sequence (but are detailed herein only where explanation is necessary). The following reference key is also applicable:

B = beginning student in clinical practicum (1st quarter)
I = intermediate student in clinical practicum (2nd quarter)
A = advanced student in clinical practicum (3rd quarter or more)
E = student in externship assignment

II. PROFESSIONAL INTERACTION	B	I	A	E
A. Approachability and responsiveness to supervisor	3	4	5	5
• participation in supervisory conferences				
• willingness to discuss supervisor's recommendations				
• adaptability to different forms of supervision				
B. Approachability and responsiveness to students/patients and patient's family	2	3	4	5
• adaptability to clininical population				
— communicative skills (re: patient's mode of communication, age, socioeconomic status, degree of hearing impairment, cultural background, other handicapping conditions)				
— acceptance (re: patient's mode of communication, age, socioeconomic status, degree of hearing impairment, cultural background, other handicapping conditions)				

	B	I	A	E
B. Approachability and Responsiveness *(continued)*				
• demonstration of appropriate concern (empathy, sincerity, sensitivity to patient's needs, nonverbal communication)				
C. Poise in professional interactions	2	3	4	5

IV. KNOWLEDGE AND APPLICATION OF TEST TECHNIQUES

	B	I	A	E
A. Conventional audiometry				
1. Giving instructions	3	4	5	5
2. Air conduction techniques	3	4	5	5
3. Bone conduction techniques	3	4	5	5
4. Speech audiometric techniques	3	4	5	5
5. Use of masking	2	3	5	5
6. Impedance audiometry	2	3	5	5

APPENDIX B.
Excerpts from Evaluation of Student in Clinical Practicum

Rate the student's professional competencies in terms of the following scale by circling the most appropriate numbers:

1 — awareness of competency not apparent
2 — awareness of competency apparent but not implemented
3 — competency emerging but not well developed
4 — competency developed but needs refinement and/or consistency
5 — competency well developed and demonstrated consistently
X — not applicable

II. PROFESSIONAL INTERACTION
A. Approachability and responsiveness to
supervisor   1 2 3 4 5 X
B. Approachability and responsiveness to
students/patients and patient's family   1 2 3 4 5 X
C. Poise in professional interactions   1 2 3 4 5 X

IV. KNOWLEDGE AND APPLICATION OF TEST TECHNIQUES:

Rate the student's knowledge of test techniques and his or her competence in applying this knowledge in clinical work in terms of the following scale:

1 **Unsatisfactory** — cannot or does not learn techniques; needs constant supervision
2 **Fair** — needs supervision on most tasks
2 **Average** — knows test techniques fairly well; requires moderate amount of supervision
4 **Good** — well informed on most aspects of testing; seldom requires assistance
5 **Excellent** — completely knowledgeable on all phases of testing
X **Not applicable**

A. Conventional audiometry (Check: Adults ☐   Children ☐)
1. Giving instructions   1 2 3 4 5 X
2. Air conduction techniques   1 2 3 4 5 X
3. Bone conduction techniques   1 2 3 4 5 X
4. Speech audiometric techniques   1 2 3 4 5 X
5. Use of masking   1 2 3 4 5 X
6. Impedance audiometry   1 2 3 4 5 X

APPENDIX C.
Grading System for Audiology Practicum

Clinical grades will be assigned according to the following criteria. In multiple-criteria categories, the grade may be based on any of the factors.

A *Criterion 1:* Surpasses significant number of goals.

Criterion 2: Shows exceptional progress in key areas of the particular clinical assignment without falling short of expected goals in other areas.

Criterion 3: Demonstrates outstanding performance in most areas of the particular clinical assignment, even though goals not necessarily surpassed. (This may occur in the case of an advanced student, the majority of whose goals are set at 4 or 5, thus making it difficult, if not impossible, for the student to surpass a significant number of them.)

AB Balanced combination of A and B criteria.

B *Criterion 1:* Meets significant number of goals; may also surpass a few goals for isolated competency items or in competency areas of secondary importance in the particular clinical assignment while falling short of few or no goals. (The latter must be positively balanced or outnumbered by goals surpassed.)

Criterion 2: Almost, but not quite, meets requirements of criterion 1, yet shows exceptional progress in some key area(s) of the particular clinical assignment.

BC Balanced combination of B and C criteria.

C *Criterion 1:* Falls short of significant number of goals; does not make satisfactory progress in key areas of the particular clinical assignment, but meets some goals of secondary importance.

F *Criterion 1:* Falls short of virtually all goals.

Criterion 2: Shows no observable progress in any competency area.

Definition of Terms
Goal: expected minimal achievement level
Significant: more than three
Exceptional, Outstanding: extraordinary in some way
Satisfactory: acceptable to supervisor

CHAPTER 3

Career Development: An Issue for the Master's Degree Supervisor

Elizabeth Gavett

Despite the fact that clinical supervisors have been part of speech–language pathology and audiology training programs for many years, only during the last decade has there been a major focus on numerous aspects of supervision. Although the supervisory process has become better understood, many uncertainties remain regarding career expectatiohs and development. Master's degree university clinical supervisors in speech–language pathology and audiology do not fit neatly into academe (Gavett, 1985). This has created problems for supervisors relative to career aspirations, rank, and promotion. An explanation of career development issues should help university supervisors in Human Communication Disorders to better understand and manage their own career development. This chapter provides such an examination through the use of career development concepts, models, and research from the field of Human Resource Management.

A HUMAN RESOURCE MANAGEMENT PERSPECTIVE OF CAREER

The term *career* varies in meaning. A noted researcher in Human Resource Management, Douglas T. Hall (1976), indicated that in popular writing, the term career usually connotes either vertical mobility or particular professions. In behavioral science writing, the term carries a broader meaning, which includes objective aspects of career, such as work behavior and jobs, as well as subjective aspects, such as attitudes and values. All these elements are part of Hall's (1976) working definition of the term career: "The career is the individually perceived sequence of attitudes and behaviors associated with work-related experiences and activities over the span of the person's life" (p. 4).

Career Stage Models

Basing their ideas on the premise that a career spans the duration of an individual's work life, many researchers study career development using career stage models that coordinate events in an individual's work life with the individual's age. Although career stage models differ in the names of the stages and in the age range, they generally relate stages to a period of exploration, a period of growth, a period of stability, and a subsequent decline and withdrawal from the work environment (Hall, 1976). Career stage models are valuable in that they describe general trends or traditional work patterns and provide a framework for discussion and research. One career stage model has described progressive work or occupational stages, including a preparatory work period, an initial work period, a trial work period, a stable work period, and retirement (Miller & Form, 1951). Another model described work stages relative to developmental work processes rather than job behaviors and included the stages of growth, exploration, establishment, maintenance, and decline (Super et al., 1957).

Is there merit to the concept of career stages? Do employees actually pass through discrete stages that can be documented? Research conducted to examine the needs of young management-level employees provided evidence to support the concept that people do pass through career stages (Hall & Nougaim, 1968). These authors found the initial period of employment to be a time when people are concerned with being safe, gaining recognition, and establishing themselves in a profession or organization. During this time, individuals need to define the structure of their positions and feel secure in them as they seek to become integrated into the system. Subsequently, they become less concerned with safety and more concerned with promotion and achievement; at this second stage, individuals are less concerned with moving *into* the organization and more concerned with moving *upward* in the organization. Because the Hall and Nougaim study followed employees for only 5 years, later career stages were speculative in nature. The authors' impressions were that once employees perceive that they have achieved as much as they can within the organization, the career would level off and new interests would emerge. The authors described the initial phase as being characterized by safety concerns, the second phase by achievement needs, and the third phase by self-actualization needs.

Hall (1976) has synthesized different career stages in graphic form (see Fig. 3–1). For the purpose of subsequent discussions, Hall's career curve, indicating the relationship between career stages and career development, will serve as a reference point.

Career Stages

Four stages in career development have been charted in Figure 3–1. Levels of performance on a low-to-high scale are noted, along with approximate ages when the stages typically occur.

Exploration and Trial

Career development does not begin with one's first full-time job. Early family and educational experiences are likely to affect a person's choice of career. In addition, schooling and training may help the

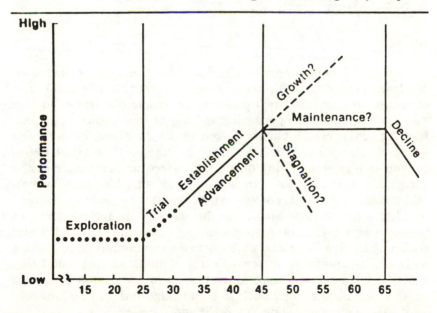

Figure 3–1. Different stages in career development. From Hall, D. T. (1976). *Careers in organizations.* Pacific Palisades, CA: Goodyear Publishing Company, Inc.

individual develop the skills needed to perform the future job tasks. It is reasonable to assume that as individuals learn work skills, they also form expectations of a particular job or career. Expectations may be influenced by family, society, or role models and may include envisioning the challenges to be faced, the rewards to be earned, the salary to be earned, the partnerships to be established, and the promotions to be achieved. When schooling and training are completed, people seek employment. When a person accepts a job, the trial phase allows time for reality testing, orientation to the organization, technical and supervisory training, and socialization (London & Stumpf, 1982). After a period of time in a first job, individuals may change organizations and repeat the trial phase, or they may remain with the organization and aspire to move up the career ladder.

Establishment and Advancement

During this career stage, individuals seek to advance within the organization, having been socialized within the system. To become established and gain advancement, people become involved in activities that lead to visibility at higher organizational levels. It becomes important to develop a level of expertise that is valued by the organization. In addition, promotions are sought at this career stage (London & Stumpf, 1982).

Mid-Career

During the mid-career stage, individuals may seek increased challenges and receive further promotions, maintain a general level of performance, or lower their performance. People who fear stagnation may strive for greater responsibility and higher status, whereas persons who fear change may choose to remain in the same job with few changes in responsibilities (London & Stumpf, 1982). Hall (1976) cautioned against assuming that a mid-career maintenance mode is necessarily a tranquil time. In fact, he noted that for some persons, mid-career can be a more stressful time than the earlier career stages. Mid-life issues that can surface at this career stage include contemplating a new career, becoming aware of advancing age and death, searching for new life goals, adapting to different family relationships and patterns, and facing a growing sense of obsolescence (Hall, 1976). Individuals who are labeled as surplus, who are demoted, or who begin to feel obsolete face decline at this stage and may be forced to seek early retirement (London & Stumpf, 1982).

Disengagement

People eventually disengage from work through the patterns of retirement, and the challenges at this stage vary. Individuals may retire either suddenly or gradually. Some persons are excited by the prospect of having time to devote to other life interests, whereas others prefer to remain active in the work force as long as possible. Learning to accept a reduced role and finding new out-of-work interests may be problematic for those who have experienced continuous growth throughout most of their careers (London & Stumpf, 1982).

APPLICATION OF THE CAREER GROWTH CURVE TO THE TRADITIONAL ACADEMICIAN

This theoretical model of career growth can easily be applied to the career path of the traditional academician. During the exploration phase, a person chooses career options and formulates job expectations based on personal values as well as on experiences. During the person's doctoral studies, important observations about life in the academic world are made. The doctoral student begins to recognize the many demands on a professor's time beyond the traditional teaching and research responsibilities. In addition, the student gains an in-depth knowledge of research expectations. Once the student completes his or her studies and joins academe, he or she probably accepts a position as an assistant professor. During this trail phase, the individual develops a self-image as a faculty member and begins to master the tasks (e.g., lecturing, grant writing, conducting research, advising students) of the job. During this time, the assistant professor becomes socialized within a new environment, both at the departmental as well as at the college and university level. Individuals learn employers' expectations and form collegial partnerships. At this career stage, an important need seems to be safety or security (Hall & Nougaim, 1968). When the person feels comfortable in the organization, and understands the job expectations, goals can be set. If persons do not sense that tenure is possible, they may move to another institution and begin the trial phase again, or they may leave academe altogether. If they believe that tenure is possible, they usually try to achieve it.

During establishment and advancement, the individual usually feels comfortable with the organization, and the need for achievement usually exceeds the need for safety (Hall & Nougaim, 1968). Career strategies must be formulated to ensure tenure and promotion.

At this time, the individual needs to become visible at higher levels within the university structure. This can be accomplished, for example, by assuming key committee positions within the university, increasing scholarly productivity, or conducting funded research. Once tenure and associate professorship are attained, the individual moves into the next career phase, that of mid-career.

During the mid-career stage, several choices emerge. The associate professor who seeks further advancement will engage in activities that lead to full professorship. Another choice is to maintain the performance level but to engage in activities that provide other rewards, such as mentoring young faculty members or becoming involved with activities outside the work environment. A common pattern for males is to become more family oriented once they feel comfortable and achieve success in their work setting (Sheehy, 1974). Some individuals face decline at this stage. As mentioned earlier, career encompasses job tasks as well as personal values. It is reasonable to assume that the rigorous realities of today's tenure struggles may leave some persons bitter, which, in turn, may result in a decrease in productivity. Furthermore, economic factors can bring about a decline curve at this stage. Individuals whose departments are being phased out may experience obsolescence and a decrease in productivity. Some individuals will change careers and re-enter the trial phase.

Among those professors who retire from the university, some do so early in order to devote time to family and other noncareer interests. Others will retire at the expected age. Still others will stay involved in academic affairs, seek professor emeritus status, and remain active in research activities and professional organizations.

APPLICATION OF THE CAREER STAGE MODEL
TO THE MASTER'S DEGREE CLINICAL SUPERVISOR

Mapping a typical career path for the master's degree clinical supervisor in Human Communication Disorders is more difficult than mapping a typical career path for the academic faculty member because of the marked inconsistency nationwide with respect to university supervisory positions. In some universities, the supervisor is in a nonacademic staff position with no obvious career ladder. Some supervisors hold academic rank but are judged by the same performance criteria used for academic faculty. Still other universities grant supervisors clinical academic ranking (e.g., clinical instructor, clinical assistant professor) and opportunity for promotion but not for tenure. As a group, supervisors lack a well-documented and established career path for which to aspire and plan.

Although supervisors are not a homogeneous group, Pickering (1985) highlighted characteristics of sex, age, and experience that probably describe a majority of clinical supervisor in Human Communication Disorders. She formulated a hypothetical job description that sought a female between the ages of 26 and 32 years (or slightly older) with 3 to 5 years of paid clinical experience. Such an individual is likely to have had some supervisory experience (probably of students in field practica sites) and some education and training in the supervisory process. It is likely that this is the individual's first full-time professional position in a university. For the purpose of discussing potential career development issues, the characteristics just noted will be considered typical of the new master's degree university supervisor.

Exploration and Trial

The exploration phase of an individual's career influences career expectations and allows for the development of job skills. Although all supervisors have been clinicans, it seems reasonable to assume that during a graduate program, students have focused on becoming competent clinicians, not competent supervisors. A student might envision a future position as a clinical supervisor, but that probably is not a primary goal. The primary aims during school are learning clinical skills, developing a self-image as a clinician, and formulating expectations of job settings such as public schools, hospitals, or private clinics. After several years as a clinician, the person decides to make a transition to supervisor. Thus, after several years in a trial phase, the individual decides to take on a new role in a new organization and repeat certain aspects of the trial phase.

After a clinician accepts the position of supervisor, she must become oriented to a new organization and develop and demonstrate new job competencies. As Hall and Nougaim (1968) pointed out in their study of young managers, safety concerns are characteristic during the early career stage. People are concerned with defining the structure of their positions, seeking security in the position, and becoming integrated into the new system. For the clinical supervisor, this means developing the self-image of a supervisor, gaining an understanding of the many tasks that must be performed, becoming comfortable in academe, and becoming aware of the university's structure.

During the trial stage of the career, individuals also face numerous challenges and conflicts. Among those faced by young managers are conflicting job expectations, insensitivity to the political environment, conflicts with an immediate work supervisor, ignorance of real evaluative criteria, loyalty dilemmas, personal anxiety, and ethical dilemmas

(Webber, 1976). New university supervisors probably experience similar challenges and conflicts. The following discussion details five of the challenges encountered by new supervisors.

Job Expectatons and Job Realities

Studies in management indicate that unrealistic job previews can lead to job dissatisfaction, whereas realistic job previews actually tend to increase job satisfaction and reduce job turnover (Wanous, 1978). If realistic job previews are important, it follows that the person best able to provide a job preview to a prospective employee is someone who is already engaged in that work. For the supervisor, that would be an individual actively involved in clinical supervision, someone who is able to interpret the published job description. Unfortunately, the persons who often provide the preview are department chairpersons or academic faculty with little or no experience in clinical supervision.

When supervisors get together, they frequently cite workload, time demands, and prestige as areas in which job expectations and job realities differ. Job previews typically identify the work as involving the direct supervision of students' clinical sessions, including observations and conferences. In addition to this primary job task, supervisors learn that they also are expected to direct and monitor general clinical management, procure and maintain field placement sites, ensure students' compliance with ASHA clinical hours requirements, and participate in department or college governance. Supervisors also frequently provide emotional support for students (Gavett, 1985). Perhaps because supervisors are physically present more often than academic faculty, or perhaps for other reasons, students often approach supervisors with their fears, insecurities, frustrations, and tears. Although such supervisor–student interactions can have a positive effect on student morale, they are time consuming for the supervisor.

There are many unpredictable day-to-day occurrences that place significant demands on a supervisor's time and cause the most efficiently planned observation and conference schedule to be altered at a moment's notice. An unexpected telephone call from a prospective client, a lengthy conversation with a field placement supervisor who is experiencing difficulty with a student, and a talk with a student in crisis are just three of the numerous unscheduled and time-consuming activities in which supervisors engage. Conflict can result when supervisors find that there is insufficient time to perform competently the job for which they were hired, namely, supervising students.

Clinicians generally regard the position of university clinical supervisor as prestigious and highly desirable. The university environment is viewed as stimulating and challenging, and supervision is viewed as a welcome change from full-time clinical activity. Furthermore, because the career ladder in the typical clinical setting is so limited, university supervisor positions allow for a career change, but one within the field. Nevertheless, what is regarded by the supervisor and her clinician colleagues as a prestigious position may not be regarded as such by the supervisor's academic colleagues at the university. Supervisors state that they sometimes feel like second-class citizens in academe. Such feelings are an unexpected part of the job reality.

The University's Political Environment

During the trial stage, the supervisor begins to learn the politics and policies of academe, many of which do not work in favor of the supervisor. Perhaps the most significant political reality that the master's degree supervisor needs to reconcile is that she has entered an environment in which the doctorate is the union card. The ramifications of not having a doctorate vary from institution to institution but typically include limited career advancement and restricted departmental involvement. The career ladder for the clinical supervisor, in fact, may have only one rung (Rassi, 1985). Frustrations expressed by supervisors frequently have to do with their lack of inclusion in department matters. Academic and clinical faculty members seldom share equally in the departmental decision-making, even though professional preparation for this field requires both didactic and clinical education.

Another political reality that supervisors face is that the structure of some universities dictates that clinical personnel have staff status rather than academic rank. An obvious advantage to staff appointment status is that it can protect against mandatory tenure review for supervisors. Staff status, however, inappropriately categorizes the job of clinical teaching. In addition, such status differentiates persons holding the positions from their appropriate peers, namely, the academic faculty.

Inappropriate or Ineffective Immediate Work Supervisor

An employee's immediate work supervisor can play an important role in the employee's development. A work supervisor can enhance the career development of a new employee by providing guidance, fostering growth opportunities, and rewarding efforts. For the clinical supervisor, the immediate work supervisor may be the department chairperson, the director of the clinic, or the clinical supervisor senior in rank. Department chairpersons, although in positions to enhance certain aspects of career development, may not be in positions to assist the clinical supervisors with day-to-day tasks because they have never been actively involved with clinical supervision or because their understanding of the job demands may be limited. Clinic directors or senior clinical supervisors may be more appropriate work supervisors because of their understanding of clinical teaching responsibilities, but they may not be in positions of influence that could facilitate growth within the organization.

Real Performance Criteria

Because "publish or perish" is not a new idea in academic institutions, supervisors are likely to be aware of this fact of academic life before they enter the university. But knowing about it as an outsider and living with it as an insider can be very different experiences. Supervisors enter the university expecting to devote their energies to supervising and teaching students. Once they arrive, they learn that excellence in clinical and academic teaching is valued and strived for but, ironically, not always rewarded. On the other hand, published research brings unequivocal documented acclaim to the academic institution. Faculty with respected research records are likely to seek and be awarded grant funds that result in increased research time, additional publications, and continued acclaim within the university. Institutional awards are usually given to those individuals who do what the university values. In academe, tenure, promotion, and merit pay are rewards for faculty; usually criteria for these institutional rewards emphasize research and grant funding. Although responsible educators strive for and value rigorous teaching standards, the reality is that during performance review, expertise in clinical and academic teaching is not as valued as grant funding and publications. In recent years, some universities have developed guidelines for merit pay that specify point values for different activities. Point values are typically higher for research and grant activities than for teaching and service activities, thus placing the clinical supervisor at an obvious disadvantage. Once supervisors become aware of academe's performance criteria, they are faced with reconciling the difference between personal and institutional values.

Ethical and Personal Dilemmas

Supervisors are legally and ethically responsible for the clients receiving treatment under their supervision. The need to procure malpractice insurance, either by the university or by the individual supervisor, is a concrete reminder of the supervisor's legal responsibilities to the clients her students treat. Current ASHA ESB accreditation standards indicate that the first 25 hours of practicum be monitored by university personnel. Beginning students in practicum often require significant involvement from the supervisor. If supervisors believe that providing extra time for students will result in positive treatment outcome for their clients, they usually provide that extra time. Supervisors often struggle with determining how much time is enough.

Another dilemma that supervisors face concerns the student who is doing poorly in clinical practicum. Failing a student in clinic usually means preventing the student from progressing in the chosen profession. Such a decision, even though it is based on clear evaluative criteria, is a difficult one and is usually not made without considerable deliberation and collegial discussion.

Another dilemma concerns referring students for counseling. This is a delicate and sensitive matter, and one with which supervisors are often confronted. Students face issues in their personal lives that may not be problematic in terms of their classroom performance but that may affect their clinical work. Supervisors must decide whether to refer, when, and how to so so. They must accept that counseling referrals are an ongoing, although difficult, part of their total responsibilities.

During this exploration and trial stage, many supervisors face the dilemma of what to do about their careers. Generally, three scenarios unfold. Some supervisors decide to pursue a doctorate. Other supervisors might leave the university or the profession. Others might remain in the position and seek continued career growth. They then would move into the establishment and advancement stage.

The reasons that a supervisor might seek a doctorate vary. Decisions might range from the desire to advance the knowledge and skill base to the recognition that a doctorate is necessary in order to remain in the academic world. A doctorate allows for increased credibility in academe and in the professional world. Securing a doctorate allows the individual not only to remain in academe and continue supervising but also to teach academic courses and have a greater voice in curriculum and departmental matters. The doctorate can allow for increased flexibility, opportunities, and options.

Some supervisors leave the university and, at times, the profession. Some supervisory positions may be defined as three- to five-year positions so that the supervisor has no say in the matter. When supervisors voluntarily leave the university or the profession, "burnout" is frequently cited as the reason. If institutional constraints dictate heavy workloads with no formal mechanism for recognition or advancement, and if individuals believe that their contributions are not valued, burnout can result. A recent ASHE-ERIC publication, *Burnout: The New Academic Disease,* described a scene that is becoming common-place in academe and one that fits the experiences of some clinical supervisors.

> A highly talented and enthusiastic individual is hired to perform a par-ticular job. Having demonstrated success at that job, other tasks and responsibilities are assigned or accepted. As financial conditions worsen, responsibilities continue to expand while support staff and services shrink. Frustration builds as the individual is no longer able to achieve the level of excellence once considered normal. Finally, exhausted from working long hours, new patterns of behavior emerge in order to face a job that is no longer enjoyable. Eventually, the individual either quits or develops a coping mentality and work pattern that make survival possible until retirement. In short, the individual's enthusiasm and commitment have burned out. (Fife, 1983 — Foreword)

The initial years of supervision are described by supervisors as highly challenging and rewarding. Nevertheless, if the demands become too great and the rewards too meager, the individual may have no choice but to leave the system.

Establishment and Advancement

What happens to the supervisor who chooses to remain in the university and seeks continued career growth? Suppose this super-visor has been challenged and rewarded, and she sees growth poten-tial within herself and within the institution. Goals during the establishment and advancement stage include seeking visibility at higher organizational levels and receiving promotions (London & Stumpf, 1982). The following discussion focuses on these two goals as well as the challenges faced at this stage.

Increased Visibility

A clinical supervisor can gain increased visibility in the depart-ment, college, or univerity in numerous ways. The University of Con-necticut Department of Communication Sciences (1986) has developed a list of activities that can facilitate career growth. These activities, which provide guidelines for nontenure track merit raise recommen-dations, are categorized by the traditional academic headings of scholarship, teaching, and service (see Appendix A).

SCHOLARSHIP. The scholarly activities in which the master's degree clinical supervisor is likely to engage differ from those in which the traditional academician is likely to engage, although there may be overlap. The traditional academician may be more likely than the typical clinical supervisor to serve as an editorial consultant and to seek grant funding. For supervisors, however, there are numerous opportunities to make scholarly presentations and to publish. For example, supervisors who are recognized as experts in a particular clinical disorder area or a particular aspect of supervision may present workshops at the local, state, and national levels. Furthermore, depending on the area of expertise, supervisors may submit or be invited to submit articles, technical reports, clinical or supervisory materials, chapters, or even books for publication.

TEACHING. A supervisor may gain visibility at higher organizational levels by expanding teaching activities beyond traditional one-to-one supervisor–student interaction. Guest lectures may be conducted within as well as outside the department. Lectures by speech-language pathologists can complement study in allied health fields, special education, child development, and other related areas. Development of innovative teaching materials and implementation of innovative approaches to supervision are other activities that can gain recognition for the supervisor.

SERVICE. There are numerous service opportunities available to the clinical supervisor. In addition to department, college, and university committees, supervisors can become involved with their state associations. On a national level, there are numerous opportunities to serve in varying capacities for ASHA and Council of University Supervisors of Practicum in Speech–Language Pathology and Audiology (CUSPSPA). All of these can be both personally and professionally rewarding.

Promotions

One characteristic of the establishment and advancement stage is the receiving of promotions. If promotion opportunities are unavailable within the university, supervisors can continue to develop their careers in other ways. London and Stumpf (1982) pointed out that career progression includes not only promotions and higher pay but also work-role changes that lead to individual growth. A work-role change that provides greater job or life satisfaction, increased sense of self-worth, and feelings of competence and achievement can be considered career progression. Supervisors who have mastered one aspect of the job can seek challenges that lead to an increase in job satisfaction and self-worth. For example, supervisors may want to increase their clinical expertise in a disorder area or learn skills in marketing or administration. In Appendix A, many areas of potential involvement for supervisors are listed.

Challenges

Challenges that might face the clinical supervisor at this career stage are different than those faced at an earlier stage. At this stage, presumably the supervisor is comfortable with her role and her environment and is becoming increasingly competent in the task she was hired to perform, that is, supervision. She has reconciled conflicts between job expectations and job realities, become aware of the university's political environment, formed positive relationships with colleagues or work supervisors, become aware of real performance criteria, and become comfortable in difficult decision-making matters. Nevertheless, she is getting further and further away from her own days as a practicing clinician. This dilemma, a frequently expressed concern of supervisors, can be addressed in various ways. For example, some individuals may provide demonstration therapy in the clinic or begin a private practice.

Institutional constraints are a second potential challenge for the supervisor at this time. It is possible that the individual is gaining visibility and exposure from her involvement in activities that are increasing her work satisfaction, but the department's needs cannot be met simultaneously. If the institutional needs prevent her from achieving additional growth, she may choose to leave the position or the profession, or she may attempt to negotiate with the institution (dean, department chairperson, or clinic director) to determine whether any accommodations can be made.

At this career phase, if not at the preceding phase, institutional constraints and requirements, as well as personal goals, may influence a person's choice to pursue doctoral studies. In some institutions, supervisors are expected to earn a doctorate in order to remain in academe. As master's level supervisors become more involved in various scholarly activities, they may realize that the doctoral degree is necessary to attain their research goals.

Mid-Career and Disengagement

Mid-career goals vary among people. It is reasonable to assume that some persons will value growth and achievement and continue to be productive in the work environment, whereas others, having already achieved their careers, will elect to reduce their work responsibilities and spend more time in out-of-work interests. Some individuals will gain satisfaction from fostering and guiding the career development of young supervisors entering academe. Others might seek the challenge of beginning a new career.

It is difficult to describe typical mid-career patterns for university clinical supervisors because clinical supervision as a specialty area within the field of Human Communication Disorders is relatively new. Of even greater significance is that most supervisors are women, and work patterns of women have changed significantly during the last two decades.

Traditionally, career stages generally correspond to the individual's chronological age, even though people experience different events at different ages and may repeat the career stage cycle more than once (London & Stumpf, 1982). Although there are many supervisors who fall into the typical mid-career age range of approximately 46 to 60 years, they, in fact, may not be in the mid-career stage of their work lives. Personal discussions with such women typically reveal that they have raised families during their 20s and early 30s, entered or re-entered the work force on a part-time basis, and gradually assumed full-time employment. Thus, although they are in the mid-career age range, they may be involved in many of the activities that better typify the establishment and advancement stage. It is interesting to speculate on patterns that may emerge in the next decade as the specialty area of clinical supervision becomes more established and as women who have been working full-time as supervisors since their mid-20s reach the typical mid-career age range.

As noted earlier, the mid-career stage may not be a tranquil time (Hall, 1976). Furthermore, the mid-career supervisor who did not maintain currency in clinical skills may experience a feeling of obsolescence. A declining performance or institutional economic pressures may force an individual at this stage to seek early retirement.

During the disengagement stage, individuals' work efforts typically decline, and they retire. Clinical supervisors, like others at this stage, may decide to leave the university to become involved in non-career interests, whereas others might choose to maintain a level of activity in academic and professional affairs.

THE MENTOR RELATIONSHIP

Any discussion on career development needs to address mentoring because of its importance in enhancing or facilitating the growth of a protégé's career. Mentoring and its benefits have been discussed extensively in the human resource management literature (Kram, 1985; Shapiro, Haseltine & Rowe, 1978; Zey, 1984). Zey (1984) defined a mentor as a person who oversees the career and development of another person, usually a junior. This person performs different functions, potentially acting as teacher, counselor, intervenor, and sponsor. As a teacher, the mentor shares information with the protégé. As a counselor, the mentor provides psychological support for the protégé. As an intervenor, the mentor protects the protégé, and, as a sponsor, the mentor either promotes or influences others to promote the protégé.

Kram (1985) described similar mentoring functions but categorized them as either career functions or psychosocial functions. She defined the former as those activities that facilitate advancement in the organization and that assist the protégé to learn about the organization, gain exposure, receive promotions, be assigned challenging work, and feel protected. Thus, the protégé's sense of competence, identity, and effectiveness is enhanced. Psychosocial functions include providing role-modeling, acceptance, confirmation, counseling, and friendship.

Shapiro and colleagues (1978) also acknowledged the benefits of mentoring. They suggested that different types of career support and guidance are provided by different individuals within an organization. They suggested a continuum with "mentor" at one end and "peer–pal" at the other end. Their view is that whereas mentor-protégé dyads tend toward being hierarchical, parental, and elitist, relationships that fall toward the peer–pal end of the continuum are significantly less so. Although the peer relationship may not result in the same career mobility as a mentor relationship, it provides important support and guidance.

Mentoring relationships are dynamic and change over time as individuals pass through different career stages and as needs change. Kram (1985) described four predictable phases of a mentoring relationship as well as characteristics associated with each phase. Her research is based on interviews with 18 pairs of managers involved in developmental work relationships in a corporate work setting. (The group of protégés included 10 male and 8 female subjects and the group of mentors included 17 males and 1 female.)

Phases of Mentoring

The first phase of mentoring, initiation, usually involves the first 6 to 12 months of the relationship. During this time, both individuals mutually select one another. The senior member of the pair is respected for his or her competence and ability to provide support. The junior member is someone who welcomes being coached and supported.

The next phase described by Kram, cultivation, lasts from two to five years and is the phase during which the relationship reaches its peak. Both career-building activities and psychosocial support may be provided during this phase. The degree to which the senior partner can help the protégé build his or her career depends somewhat on the senior's rank and influence in the organization. The degree of trust between the two persons usually determines the extent of psychosocial support provided. It is during this cultivation phase that the relationship evolves from being one-sided to being more mutually beneficial. As the protégé becomes increasingly skillful and develops confidence, he or she is able to give to the mentor. In addition, the mentor is rewarded by seeing the protégé move up the career ladder.

The third phase, separation, usually occurs after two to five years in the cultivation stage, or when the individual's needs or the organizational circumstances change. The protégé no longer may need guidance or support from the mentor. Job changes or promotions within the organization can create a distance between the two people or force a separation. Individuals often feel a sense of turmoil and loss during the separation phase. Mentoring functions change during this phase; some may no longer be necessary; others may be modified. This important phase allows the protégé to perform successfully without the mentor's support and allows the mentor to acknowledge success in facilitating a new talent.

After separation is accepted, the fourth and final phase, redefinition, can occur. Although relationships can be redefined to provide differing kinds of career or psychosocial support, Kram (1985) found that friendship typically characterizes this phase. Some relationships at this phase may be redefined to mean absence of contact. If the psychosocial functions had been minimal or absent, this latter pattern would be the one more likely to have taken place.

The Female Protégé

Because the hypothetical description of the typical clinical supervisor is one who is female, it is relevant to identify potential barriers to women as protégés. Despite the fact that women in managerial positions are increasing in number, there are indications that they continue to face gender-related barriers that can inhibit career progression within an organization (Zey, 1984). Men and women have indicated that sexual tension and fear of increasing intimacy can lead to anxiety and confusion in a cross-gender relationship (Kram, 1985).

Men and women may be reluctant to cultivate a strong mentoring relationship because of the threat of sexual attraction. Although Zey (1984) acknowledged the sexual issue as a barrier to male–female mentor relationships, he viewed women's relatively weak status in the work world as a more significant obstacle. A mentor is likely to choose a protégé who is highly likely to succeed. If the organization does not promote women readily, they are less likely to be selected as protégés. Zey expressed optimism about changes for women in management positions. As numbers of women in managerial positions increase, male–female partnerships should be more commonplace.

Mentoring in Academe

It is reasonable to assume that academic mentoring occurs. Discussing career mobility for the traditional academician, Carter (1982) argued that a mentor relationship not only was desirable but also was necessary. She pointed out that this is particularly true for minority individuals and women. Zey's (1984) view that women's relatively weak status in the work environment is a major obstacle to forming mentor relationships seems to be particularly relevant when discussing clinical supervisors in academe. If mentors choose protégés who are highly likely to succeed in that organization, a presumption has been made that the organization allows for the growth and promotion of that protégé. This is not always true for clinical supervisors.

ENHANCING THE CLINICAL SUPERVISOR'S CAREER GROWTH

Given what the field of Human Resources Management suggests about career development, supervisors who are interested in enhancing their own career growth might focus energy in three areas: (1) reducing the university's organizational constraints, (2) establishing mentor relationships, and (3) understanding career development issues specific to supervision.

Reducing Organizational Constraints

A university's organizational policies present certain career barriers for the master's degree clinical supervisor. Although institutions vary, academe is usually comprised of persons who hold the doctorate degree and whose primary responsibilities are academic teaching and research. Thus, academic policies and requirements reflect the needs of these individuals. Nevertheless, because clinical training programs do exist in universities, universities need to acknowledge the difference between academic and clinical teaching and to accommodate fully those persons involved in clinical teaching. One major organizational issue that must be clarified concerns the degree expected of clinical teachers. A second major issue concerns career advancement opportunities. Regardless of degree, clinical supervisors in some institutions are unable to advance because the system's criteria for advancement are inappropriate for the clinical teacher. Supervisors and their academic colleagues are left to work within the organization to reduce various constraints.

Establishing Mentor Relationships

Mentor and peer relationships provide support and guidance for young employees in many work settings. Master's degree clinical supervisors would benefit greatly from support during their first years in the university. Experienced clinical supervisors and senior academic faculty members would be appropriate persons to provide such guidance. These individuals could help the supervisor become aware of the university's political structure and real performance criteria and assist in establishing goals. They may also be able to provide opportunities for the supervisor to assist them in scholarly activities.

Supervisors need to recognize the important role that a mentor can play in career development and seek such support. When mentors are not available in the organization, supervisors can look to other sources; for example, CUSPSPA serves as an excellent resource for such peer support.

Understanding Career Development Issues

There is little or no preparation in career development in our professional training programs. To students in Human Communication Disorders, career development issues drawn from business management may seem to have little in common with human service delivery. This is not true. In fact, the field of Organizational Behavior may be an important resource for clinical supervisors striving to understand and become active participants in their own career development.

CONCLUSION

Considerable literature exists on the work lives of men and their careers in business and industry. This is not true for the work lives and careers of university supervisors in speech–language pathology and audiology, who are primarily women. This chapter has drawn from literature that is primarily about men's careers in order to discuss and speculate on various career issues that master's degree clinical supervisors face in academe. As the specialty area of supervision continues to develop and as its research base increases, attention needs to be focused on those individuals who provide these services, on the challenges that they confront, and on the career opportunities available to them. Gender, degree status, institutional policies, and type of teaching activity are some of the variables that can and do influence the careers of clinical supervisors. It is time for these professional issues to be examined systematically.

REFERENCES

Carter, H. (1982). Making it in academia: Gurus can get you there? In *The academic mentor: Guru, gatekeeper or guide.* Symposium conducted at the meeting of the Educational Research Association, New York.

Fife, J. (1983). Foreword. In W. A. Melendez & R. M. Guzman (Eds.), *Burnout: he new academic disease.* ASHE-ERIC Higher Education Research Report No. 9, Washington, DC: Association for the Study of Higher Education.

Gavett, E. (1985). Competence, qualifications, training: Speech–language pathology. In J. E. Bernthal (Ed.), *Proceedings of the Sixth Annual Conference on Graduate Education* (pp. 20–25). Lincoln, NE: University of Nebraska, Council of Graduate Programs in Communication Sciences and Disorders.

Hall, D. T. (1976). *Careers in organizations.* Pacific Palisades, CA: Goodyear Publishing.

Hall, D. T. & Nougaim, K. E. (1968). An examination of Maslow's need hierarchy in an organizational setting. *Organizational Behavior and Human Performance, 3,* 12–35.

Kram, K. E. (1985). *Mentoring at work.* Glenview, IL: Scott, Foresman.

London, M. & Stumpf, S. A. (1982). *Managing careers.* Reading, MA: Addison-Wesley Publishing.

Miller, D. C. & Form, W. H. (1951). *Industrial society.* New York: Harper & Bros.

Pickering, M. (1985). Clinical supervision in a university setting: Overview of the topic. In J. E. Bernthal (Ed.), *Proceedings of the Sixth Annual Conference on Graduate Education* (pp. 15–19). Lincoln, NE: University of Nebraska, Council of Graduate Programs in Communication Sciences and Disorders.

Rassi, J. (1985). Competencies, qualifications, training: Audiology. In J. E. Bernthal (Ed.), *Proceedings of the Sixth Annual Conference on Graduate Education* (pp. 26–32). Lincoln, NE: University of Nebraska, Council of Graduate Programs in Communication Sciences and Disorders.

Shapiro, E. C., Haseltine, F. P. & Rowe, M. P. (1978). Moving up: Role models, mentors and the patron system. *Sloan Management Review, 10,* 51–88.

Sheehy, G. (1974). *Passages.* New York: E. P. Dutton.

Super, D., Crites, J., Hummel, R., Moser, H., Overstreet, P. & Warrath, C. (1957). *Vocational development: A framework for research.* New York: Teachers College Press.

University of Connecticut, Department of Communication Sciences. (1986). *Guidelines for merit raise recommendations: Non-tenure track.* Unpublished chart.

Wanous, J. P. (1978). Realistic job previews: Can a procedure to reduce turnover also influence the relationship between abilities and performance? *Personnel Psychology, 31*(2), 249–258.

Webber, R. A. (1976). Career problems of young managers. *California Management Review, 18*(4), 19–33.

Zey, M. (1984). *The mentor connection.* Homewood, IL: Dow Jones-Irwin.

APPENDIX A.
The University of Connecticut Guidelines for Merit Raise Recommendations Nontenure Track
January 31, 1986

I. Scholarship
  A. Scholarly presentations   5–20
     National
     Out-of-state
     State-wide
     Local
     Adjustments determined by nature of presentation (invited, contributed, panel, multiauthor, and so on), length of presentation (3-day vs. 1-hour), size and nature of group.
  B. Grants and Contracts
     Federal
       Funded   40
       Approved without funding   25
       Not approved   15
     University Research Foundations   5–15
     Other (explain)
     Adjustments determined by factors such as principal vs. co-investigator, amount of funding, proposed budget, and so on.
  C. Editorial Consultant   10–20
     Adjustment determined by nature of publication, responsibilities of appointment, and so on.
  D. Publications
     Books
       Authored   50
       Edited   40
     Articles
       Refereed   35
       Nonrefered (including book reviews)   15
     Technical Reports   10
     Adjustments made on the basis of single vs. multiauthor, senior author vs. co-author, scope and distribution of publication, and so on.
  E. Other

II. Teaching
    A. Supervisory rating   5–10
    B. Innovative supervisory practices   5–20
    Adjustments will be based on the nature of the activity and expected impact or demonstrated result.
    C. Innovative clinical procedures   5–20
    Adjustments will be based on the nature of the activity and expected impact or demonstrated result.
    D. Departmental lectures or other teaching   1–25
    Adjustments will be based on length and nature of the teaching.
    E. Extent and nature of supervisory or clinical workload   1–10
    Adjustments will be made for unusual circumstances, such as continuing overloads, new responsibilities, and so on, which are not otherwise compensated.
    F. Academic advising   1–5
    G. Other
III. Service
    A. Departmental committees, including NSSLHA
        Chair or Advisor   3–10
        Member   1–5
    B. University or AAUP committees
        Chair   5–12
        Member   5–7
    C. Professional organizations
        Office
            National   8–30
            State   5–20
            Local   1–5
        Committee
            National   5–15
            State   3–10
            Local   1–3
    Adjustments determined by nature of organization and position (e.g., type of office, committee chair vs. committee member).
    D. Outreach   1–10
    Outreach is defined as performing for no extra compensation a function for the department as a result of contractual arrangements made by the department (UCHC, LEAs and RESCs, VNAs, nursing homes, and so on). Also, any other functions not listed elsewhere that enhance the status of the department.

III. Service (*continued*)
    E. CFY Supervision   5
    F. Other
IV. Miscellaneous
    A. Honors and Awards   1-25
       Adjustments determined by nature and scope of the honor or award.
    B. Other

Printed with permission from the University of Connecticut Department of Communication Sciences.

PART II

Research Perspectives

CHAPTER 4

Research on Human Communication Disorders Supervision

Donald G. Doehring

T his chapter is concerned with research on Human Communication Disorders supervision. It is a representative rather than an exhaustive survey, with emphasis on recent research but attention to important earlier research. A thorough review of all research is not possible because of space limitations. Selected studies are described to illustrate the kinds of strategies that have been devised to meet the special problems of supervision research. After the survey of research, the trends are summarized (the reader may wish to begin with the summary), the research is evaluated, and suggestions are made regarding the directions of future research.

SURVEY OF SUPERVISION RESEARCH

As in all research on communication disorders, there are problems in reaching valid conclusions by using methods that were designed for basic research, but supervision researchers have been remarkably successful. Researchers have been concerned with defining the clinical skills acquired through supervision training and relating these to the characteristics of student clinicians and supervisors. Particular attention has been paid to the interaction of students and supervisors during supervisory conferences. Many of the data have been gathered by questionnaires and rating scales filled out by supervisors, student clinicians, clients, and independent raters, with considerable reliance on audiotaped and videotaped conferences. There is some indication that future research may use nonstandard research methods that recognize the special interpersonal nature of supervision,as discussed by Pickering (see chap. 5).

Research on supervision is intended to evaluate the effectiveness of current supervision practices and indicate directions for improvement. On the whole, research has been well-focused on relevant problems. The major research topics relate to characteristics of student clinicians, characteristics of supervisors, analysis of supervision conferences, comparison of supervision methods, and pretraining in clinical skills. These topics will be reviewed in that order.

Characteristics of Student Clinicians

How do the personal characteristics of students relate to their success in completing supervised practical training? Research by Shriberg and colleagues (1975) provides an example of how researchers with extensive practical experience have approached this basic question of supervision research. Their research is described here in detail. The research was carefully planned and executed, and interpreted with suitable caution. Equally important, their work illustrates some of the limitations inherent in using standard research methods for answering questions about supervision.

The first task confronting researchers who wish to assess the effects of supervision is to obtain a measure of clinical competence. This is a problem in itself, which Shriberg and his collaborators approached in a well-organized manner. They defined clinical competence on the basis of their own and their colleagues' experience to include four domains of skill: assessment, management, counseling of client and family, and interactions with other professionals. They recognized the practical difficulties of obtaining direct, objective measures of competence and accepted the necessity for assessing competence indirectly through subjective ratings of supervisors. A 38-item form was developed for appraisal of the clinical competence of students by their supervisors. This form, called the *Wisconsin Procedure for Appraisal of Clinical Competence* (W-PACC), was appropriate for different kinds of practica and different orientations to supervision. In agreement with the majority of their colleagues, the investigators differentiated two aspects of clinical competence: professional-technical skills for dealing with the client's disorder and interpersonal skills for establishing an effective working relationship with the client.

Test-retest reliability of raters was established by correlating supervisors' ratings of the same student clinician on two separate occasions a few days apart. *Split-half reliability* showing internal consistency of the form was determined by correlating the scores on odd-numbered items with the scores on even-numbered items. Both types of reliability were satisfactory for both types of tests, indicating that the forms would be consistently scored by the types of supervisors who participated in the preliminary studies.

Content validity was assessed by obtaining agreement from supervisors that the items and the scoring procedure reflected their own ways of judging clinical competence. *Construct validity* was determined by establishing that the scores on technical items correlated more highly with each other than with the scores on interpersonal items, and vice versa. (It is very important to note, however, that there was a high correlation [0.70] between professional-technical and interpersonal scores.) *Criterion validity*, the ultimate test of how well the scores on the W-PACC reflected the actual clinical competence of the student, was estimated by the correlation between scores on the W-PACC and clinical grades given the students by their supervisors. The clinical grades correlated highly with technical skills but not with interpersonal skills when the correlation between the two types of skills was partialled out. There was a suggestion that the interpersonal skills of beginning clinicians were better than their technical skills.

The next step was to determine how the personal characteristics of 239 undergraduate and graduate students, comprising six groups, were related to their clinical competence (Shriberg, Bless, Carlson, Filley, Kwiatkowski & Smith, 1977). A large number of correlations was calculated among 30 measures for the six groups. Only those of greatest relevance will be summarized here. The most consistent finding was that clinical competence was related to academic achievement. The writers, noting that previous research had demonstrated a strong relationship between intellectual ability and academic achievement, concluded that clinical competence was highly dependent on intellectual ability. The relationship of clinical competence to interest and personality measures was weaker and less consistent but suggestive. Clinical competence was associated with a high initial interest in clinical work, with the attitude that positive and negative events are under one's own control rather than determined by outside forces, with a high need for approval, and with emotional stability. Once again, a high correlation was again found between technical and interpersonal skills, but no further conclusions were reached about the differential relationship of the two types of skill to clinical grades. Clinical grades tended to remain the same from the beginning to the end of clinical training. There was little room for variation, because 94 percent of the clinical grades were either A or AB. There was no mention of change in the W-PACC scores from the beginning to the end of clinical training.

The research of Shriberg and colleagues is exemplary in several respects. It was carefully planned by teams of investigators who had an exceptional grasp of both research and supervision. A formal scale was developed for assessing clinical competence and a large number of measures were obtained for a large group of student clinicians in order to assess the relationship between personal characteristics and clinical competence. The results, which were interpreted with appropriate caution, were interesting and provocative. They suggested that bright, self-sufficient, ambitious, emotionally stable students with strong clinical interests will tend to receive the highest ratings of clinical competence, perhaps on the basis of their technical skills rather than their interpersonal skills. This is a considerable amount of useful information.

It is difficult to obtain an exact fit between the needs of practically-oriented research and the rigorous requirements of conventional research methods. Like almost all nonlaboratory research that is aimed at obtaining information of practical use, the research of Shriberg and colleagues has a number of shortcomings:

1. Despite the amount of time and effort that went into the research and the large number of measures and subjects:
   a. The findings of Shriberg and his colleagues are not definitive and "need to be replicated within other training programs" (1977, p. 320). The likelihood of other researchers going to the effort and expense involved in this research is doubtful.
   b. The practical difficulties of obtaining complete measures on all subjects prevented the researchers from determining many relationships of interest, such as the relationship of academic achievement to technical and interpersonal skills.
   c. More measures would be needed to determine other relationships of interest, such as the assessment of clinical competence within the separate skill domains.
2. Correlational research has inherent limitations. A high correlation between two measures such as academic achievement and clinical competence may not be indicative of a cause-

and-effect relationship, but rather of mutual correlation with a third variable.

3. Different results might be obtained with different measures, particularly on the personality scales and the clinical ratings.

4. When using standard research designs involving statistical tests, it is necessary to have adequate variability in the measures obtained. In the study of Shriberg and colleagues, the clinical grades showed little variability, the majority being excellent or near excellent.

5. The basic question of the effects of supervision was not directly addressed by this research.

A number of other investigations has contributed interesting and useful information about student clinicians. Oratio (1976a) obtained 382 statements from 25 different training programs regarding criteria for evaluating the speech and language therapy skills of student clinicians. Through several stages, the statements were reduced to 40 unambiguous, nonoverlapping items scored on a seven-point scale, where one was the most favorable rating. A total of 207 evaluations of student clinicians was obtained from 152 supervisors in 53 training programs. The ratings were factor-analyzed, and the two factors that emerged were interpreted as technical skills (10 items) and interpersonal skills (eight items), thus corroborating and extending the findings of Shriberg and colleagues (1975). One important feature of this study was that all data were obtained by mail. Another was that none of the 40 items had average ratings above two on the seven-point scale, confirming the genèrally high ratings of student clinicians reported by Shriberg and colleagues (1977).

It will be recalled that Shriberg and colleagues (1977) found a consistently strong relationship between technical and interpersonal skills, even though they could be differentiated. Oratio (1978a) re-analyzed the data from his 1976 study, calculating canonical correlations between technical items and interpersonal items and found a strong relationship between the two skills, again confirming the findings of Shriberg and colleagues using a different rating scale, students, supervisors, and method of statistical proof.

Oratio (1978b) next studied the relationship between the ratings of supervisors and the self-ratings of student clinicians. In a previous study, Caracciolo (1977) found that the self-ratings of advanced student clinicians were significantly higher than those of their supervisors. Oratio obtained self-ratings from beginning student clinicians and ratings from their supervisors on a 27-item scale that assessed three domains of clinical competence (technical and interpersonal skills, and target behaviors) and 2 domains of client behavior (rapport and therapy feedback) that had been identified in another large factor analytic study (Oratio, 1980). There were relatively high correlations between student and supervisor ratings for all but the technical skills, with no significant difference in the mean ratings, indicating that beginning clinicians rated all domains of competence in the same manner as their supervisors, except the skill on which the supervisors based their clinical grades (Shriberg et al., 1975). In agreement with the suggestive finding of Shriberg and colleagues (1977), there was a more favorable average rating for interpersonal skills than technical skills for these beginning clinicians.

Dowling (1984) also found that self-ratings of student clinicians did not differ significantly from ratings of supervisors and fellow students. The degree of relationship was not directly demonstrated, however, because she did not calculate the correlation among the ratings.

In another study, Dowling (1985) used a slightly different approach to study clinical competence. She classified student clinicians as outstanding, average, and failing on the basis of their supervisors' written impressions of their clinical performance. Then she had the supervisors rate the students on a 36-item checklist that covered five domains of competence: planning and report writing, therapy techniques, evaluation and reinforcement techniques, professional conduct, and personal conduct (including interpersonal relations). Outstanding students received near-perfect ratings on all items, average students received average ratings on all items, and failing students received near-minimum ratings on all but three items. This suggested that there were no particular areas of strength or weakness that could be pointed out to supervisors. In agreement with previous studies, a very small proportion of students were classified as failing, and a much larger proportion were classified as outstanding. The limitation of this study was that the use of group averages could have masked individual variability. A statistical procedure that classified students according to individual rather than group profiles (Aram & Nation, 1975) might have revealed different patterns of strengths and weaknesses among failing students, thus providing supervisors with more useful information.

A quite different result had been obtained by Dowling and Bliss (1984), who found that outstanding and failing student clinicians did not differ on two measures that were supposed to underlie interpersonal skills: cognitive complexity (complexity of interpersonal constructs) and rhetorical sensitivity (thinking about what should be said and deciding how to say it). The conflicting results in two studies involving the same investigator raise two possibilities. In the Dowling and Bliss (1984) study, the measures of interpersonal skill may have been too artificial and indirect to reflect the actual interpersonal skills of the student clinicians; or, in the Dowling (1985) study, the three groups may have differed on all items because of a "halo effect" produced by the overall judgments of supervisors regarding clinical competence. The possibilities are equally disturbing.

Sleight (1985) was concerned with students' anxieties about clinical training. She thought that students beginning in practicum might tend to be most anxious. On the basis of discussions in the literature she selected 40 items reflecting anxiety about supervisors' standards, responsibility for clients, applying theory to practice, and general practicum functioning. She found that beginning practicum students, nonpracticum students, and students doing observations were all relatively confident in all domains, with the practicum students becoming significantly more confident by the end of clinical training. Thus, anxiety does not seem to be a problem for most students at any stage of clinical training. The finding of increased confidence in advanced student clinicians agrees with Caracciolo's (1977) finding of higher self-ratings by advanced student clinicians, suggesting that, if anything, over-confidence may be a problem.

Finally, clients' opinions about student clinicians have not been neglected. Haynes and Oratio (1978) constructed a 56-item rating scale where the clients rated each statement on a seven-point scale according to its contribution to effective therapy. A total of 162 questionnaires was completed by adult clients in 48 clinical institutions nationwide. Factor-analysis resulted in seven factors. The strongest (seven items, 47 percent of total variance) was Demographic and included the clinician's age, sex, physical appearance, and race. Others were identified as Directness (four items, 19 percent), involving goal achievement and understanding, Technical Skill (three items, nine percent), Empathic Genuineness (four items, seven percent), Concreteness (three items, six percent), and Proximity (three items, five percent). In this study, the importance of factors was judged in terms of the mean ratings of the contribution to effective therapy. The highest importance was given by the clients to technical skill and empathic-genuineness items, both having mean ratings of 6.3 out of a possible seven. The demographic factor, which accounted for the most variance, was rated as least important. The items dealing with age, sex, physical appearance, and race of the clinician had a mean rating of only 2.8 out of seven. This study demonstrated that clients' perceptions of clinical competence agreed with those of supervisors and student clinicians in emphasizing technical and interpersonal skills. It also showed that the clinician's "demographic" characteristics are not as important to the client as the clinician may think they are.

These studies of clinical competence show an excellent focus on the practical issues of supervision, successful use of conventional research designs, and sophisticated statistical analyses. There was general agreement that clinical competence can be divided into technical and interpersonal skills, that most students are rated as very competent, and that the most competent students tend to be bright, stable, and well-oriented toward clinical work.

Characteristics of Supervisors

How do supervisors' characteristics relate to students' clinical competence? Schubert and Aitchison (1975) distributed a questionnaire to supervisors and received replies from 79 percent of the graduate programs in speech pathology and audiology in the United States. Of the 501 supervisors who responded, 63 percent were women, 78 percent were between the ages of 25 and 45 years, and 40 percent had less than two years' professional experience before becoming supervisors. Although 64 percent had no formal training in supervision, 83 percent thought specific academic courses in supervision would be important for supervisors. However, 91 percent believed themselves adequately prepared for supervision, and 84 percent considered their supervisory position equal or superior to a teaching position. The majority (77 percent) supervised more than five students per week and 24 percent supervised more than 15 students per week. Post-therapy conferences were used by 98 percent, 67 percent used videotaped sessions, and 72 percent used objective evaluation systems. Thus, in 1975, supervisors tended to be mature, serious about their positions, hardworking, attentive to evaluation, and not concerned about their professional status or lack of formal training.

The competence of supervisors has not been evaluated as systematically as that of student clinicians. This is not surprising, because supervisors are not supervised as closely as students. Oratio, Sugarman, and Prass (1981) reported few previous attempts to evaluate supervisors. Their review of the literature indicated that supervision involves teaching, leadership, evaluation, administration, behavioral analysis, interpersonal relations, and counseling and that the supervisor is expected to be sensitive, open-minded, genuine, resourceful, objective, rational, knowledgeable, flexible, tolerant, and able to maintain facilitative verbal interactions with student clinicians. Previous research did not support these expectations, indicating that supervisors were nonfacilitative (Irwin, 1975; Culatta & Seltzer, 1976). Oratio and colleagues wished to determine the principal components of effective supervision from the perspective of the student clinician. They prepared a 54-item rating scale that sampled six hypothesized domains (administration, instruction, communication, interpersonal, professionalism, and flexibility) that were obtained by surveying the literature and submitting preliminary versions to clinicians and student clinicians. A questionnaire containing the 54 items plus an overall rating of effectiveness was completed by 164 student clinicians from 37 clinical facilities. Each item was rated on a seven-point scale on which seven was outstanding. The results were factor analyzed, and two interpretable factors emerged. The major factor, which accounted for 59 percent of the total variance in ratings, was identified as Interpersonal and the minor factor (five percent of variance) as Administration. Oratio and colleagues perhaps over-interpreted these findings to indicate that the essence of supervision was the establishment of empathy between the supervisor and the student clinician. Further research is needed to determine why factors representing the other domains of supervisor competence did not emerge. One positive finding was that students tended to rate their supervisors toward the outstanding end of the scale on all items.

Crichton and Oratio (1984) extended research on supervisor effectiveness to include supervision during the clinical fellowship year. A questionnaire containing 47 of the items from the Oratio and colleagues' (1981) study was completed by 340 former clinical fellows. Two factors again emerged, with the major factor (54 percent of total variance) identified as Interpersonal and the minor factor (six percent) this time called Supervisory Commitment. Even when supervision occurred after the completion of clinical training, the clinical fellows shared the student clinicians' perspective regarding interpersonal relationships in rating their supervisors.

Dowling and Wittkopp (1982) studied 191 students' ratings of supervisory needs (as opposed to effectiveness) on a 43-item scale that assessed five areas (lesson plan and report writing, supervisory observation, conferencing, professional responsibility, and general supervisory practices). Empathy and rapport were not rated. There was general agreement on the desire for regular joint planning, observation, conferences, evaluative feedback, and joint responsibility for clients. Experienced students wanted more responsibility for planning, and felt more responsible for the clients' welfare. Students from different training programs differed in preferences for lesson plans or discussions, as well as attitudes toward frequency of therapy observation by supervisors.

Sleight (1984) was concerned with the abilities of supervisors to rate their own competence. She cited studies that suggested that the supervisors' perception of supervision did not agree with that of student clinicians (Culatta, Colucci & Wiggins, 1975) and that supervisors tended to rate themselves lower than the students rated them (Ulrich & Watt, 1977). She compared the self-evaluations of eight supervisors with evaluations of the supervisors by 35 student clinicians on a practicum and supervision evaluation form developed at Pennsylvania State University that rated five domains of supervision (providing information and technical support, fulfilling supervisory responsibilities, facilitating interpersonal communication, fostering student autonomy, and providing professional models). All ratings were anonymous. Five of the eight supervisors rated themselves higher than the students rated them. The supervisors' mean self-ratings were higher on 28 of the 42 items. The only domain for which self-ratings tended to be lower than student ratings was fostering student autonomy, but the supervisors also rated themselves lower on an overall rating of supervisor effectiveness. Because the actual means were not given, it is not possible to determine whether all mean ratings tended to be on the postive side of the five-point scale.These results again suggest that supervisors and students have different perspectives about supervisor effectiveness, even though they tend to agree about student competence.

Several studies have been concerned with the subjectivity and variability of supervisors' evaluations of students. Runyan and Seal (1985) asked 100 supervisors to view a five-minute videotaped segment of a language therapy session and then write 10 comments for the clinician and complete a 10-item rating scale. The comments were often contradictory. The ratings were variable, with the distributions approaching a normal probability curve for some items. There was often disagreement between the written comments and the ratings. Oratio (1976b) had 20 supervisors view a 10-minute segment of a videotaped articulation therapy session and evaluate the student clinician on Oratio's (1976a) 18-item scale of technical and interpersonal skills. Half of the supervisors were told that the student clinician was an undergraduate in the first term of practicum, and half were told that the student clinician was a graduate student in her final practicum. The graduate student ratings were significantly higher on two of the 10 technical skill items, four of the eight interpersonal skill items, and the overall score. A regression analysis indicated that 30 percent of variance in ratings was accounted for by the supervisors' preconceptions regarding the students' training. Roberts and Naremore (1983) studied supervisor preconceptions by asking 46 supervisors to imagine good or poor therapy sessions and then discuss the outcome from several perspectives. The discussions tended to center on the student clinician rather than on the supervisor or client, indicating to the authors that supervisors approach supervision with preconceived beliefs and may exhibit bias in their decision-making because of a lack of objectivity.

The supervisor described by researchers did not seem to be the confident, optimistic, methodical person who filled out Schubert and Aitchison's questionnaire or the paragon described in the literature review of Oratio and colleagues (1981) as exhibiting a wide range of professional-technical and interpersonal skills. The research on clinical competence reviewed in the previous section must be interpreted with caution because much of that research was based on supervisors' ratings. The results that question the consistency, self-rating ability, and preconceived biases of supervisors led several of the researchers (Roberts & Naremore, 1983; Runyan & Seal, 1985) to suggest the need for training supervisors.

The Supervision Conference

A large proportion of the research on supervision concerns what actually happens during a supervision conference. Again there is a reliance on ratings by independent observers of videotaped conference excerpts as well as by the conference participants. In addition to the kinds of ratings used in research on student and supervisor characteristics, there are detailed analyses of the interpersonal communication during the conference. Two types of procedure have been used for analyzing conferences (Smith & Anderson, 1982a). Low-inference systems involve the recording of specific student clinician and supervisor behaviors as they occur during the conference. High-inference systems involve the rating of supervisor and student clinician interactions for the conference as a whole and are similar to the rating systems described in the preceding sections of this chapter.

A good example of low-inference systems is one adapted by Culatta and Seltzer (1976) from Boone and Prescott (1972). A total of 12 categories of supervisor and student clinician behavior (good and bad evaluations of students, questions, suggestions about strategies, comments about therapy session, and irrelevant comments) were coded in terms of time and duration of occurrence. Randomly selected five-minute videotaped segments of conferences of 10 supervisor–graduate student pairs over a 12-week period were analyzed. Scoring was reliable. Only nine percent of responses were evaluative, with the students mostly supplying information about therapy sessions, and the supervisors mostly asking questions and suggesting therapy strategies. This interaction pattern did not vary with differences in self-reported styles of supervision (directive, non-directive, or mixed) or during the 12 weeks.

In a second study, Culatta and Seltzer (1977) had six supervisors score and then discuss five-minute videotaped segments of their own conferences over a 12-week period. All supervisors believed that the self-analysis procedure gave useful insights. Nevertheless, the same stereotyped pattern of supervisor question–student information–supervisor strategy suggestions occurred throughout the 12-week period, even though the supervisors recognized the pattern and the need for further evaluation. When conference interactions were analyzed by a low-inference system, the observed events showed a stereotyped nonevaluative pattern that did not vary among supervisors or over time.

Dowling and Shank (1981) used the Culatta-Seltzer system to compare interactions during conventional supervisory conferences and a group teaching clinic method. There were no significant differences between methods of supervision, suggesting that the same pattern occurred even when peers joined a group conference.

Smith and Anderson (1982a) developed a 60-item high-inference scale for rating individual supervisory conferences on the basis of a review of the literature. In a preliminary study the forms were completed by 112 supervisors and their conference ratings were factor-analyzed. The three major factors were Indirect Supervision (cooperative relations between student clinicians and supervisors, 56 percent of variance), Direct Supervision (supervisor dominant, 30 percent of variance), and Supervisor Preparation (13 percent of variance). A revised scale entitled Individual Supervisory Conference Rating Scale (ISCRS) was developed for a second study by selecting eight indirect supervision items, six direct supervision items, and two items for supervisory preparation to be rated on a seven-point scale. Fifteen supervisor–student pairs audiotaped conferences for three weeks and completed the ISCRS immediately following each conference. Reliability and several types of validity were established. The ratings of the student clinicians, supervisors, and trained raters were factor-analyzed separately. Factors interpreted as direct and indirect supervision emerged in each analysis, but with somewhat differing sets of items. The factor structure of the student clinicians was unrelated to that of the other raters. These findings were interpreted as reflecting slightly different perspectives regarding direct and indirect supervision. The authors suggested that student clinicians and supervisors could benefit from discussions of their different perspectives.

Brasseur and Anderson (1983) believed that indirect styles facilitate independence and direct styles are associated with supervisor control. They presented three 20-minute videotapes of simulated conferences containing 80 percent direct, 80 percent indirect, and 50 percent direct-indirect supervisor behavior, respectively, to groups of 30 supervisors, 30 graduate student clinicians, and 30 undergraduate clinicians for rating on an 18-item modification of the ISCRS. All three groups rated the 80 percent direct conference higher on direct supervision items and the remaining two simulated conferences higher on indirect supervision items. The simulated supervision styles were distinguished easily by students as well as supervisors.

Smith and Anderson (1982b) carried out an ambitious study of the interrelationships among low-inference and high-inference conference ratings and supervisor and student clinician characteristics. Only the most salient results can be given here. Data were obtained from 24 conferences, with 15 supervisor–student pairs completing the high-inference ISCRS after the conference. Three trained raters coded low-inference MOSAICS multidimensional observation system information (Weller, 1971) from audiotaped conference recordings. Direct conference ISCRS ratings were related to less participation by students, fewer questions and answers, less discussion of objectives, more discussions about methods and materials, and fewer discussions about feelings, as revealed by the MOSAICS coding. Indirect supervision ratings were associated with more questions by students, more answers and "reflexive moves" by supervisors, and more discussion of feelings. The correlations between ISCRS and MOSAICS ratings differed for supervisors and student clinicians, indicating the need for discussions of self-perceptions of conferences. The supervisors' conference ratings were correlated with the students' experience, and the frequency of students' questions was correlated with the supervisors' level of academic training. Although these results suggest important insights, more easily interpreted results might be obtained with a less complex low-inference system.

Roberts and Smith (1982) further analyzed the MOSAICS data of Smith and Anderson (1982b) according to who was speaking and when the conference took place. The data were ratios of initiative/reflexive actions, analytic/evaluation comments, diagnostic/pre-scriptive processes, complex/simple remarks, and speaker/total participation. Both participants tended to be more analytic than evaluative, diagnostic than prescriptive, reflexive than initiating, and complex than simple. Supervisors spoke more often than students but students made more diagnostic/prescriptive comments than supervisors. The patterns did not change over three conferences. These findings agreed with those of Culatta and Seltzer (1976, 1977) in suggesting a stereotyped pattern of simple, non-evaluative supervisor-directed conferences, with the student clinician supplying diagnostic information. The writers concluded that their results did not confirm the Clinical Supervision Model of Anderson (1981), which postulated complex interactions involving equal participation in both analysis and evaluation, and questioned whether the student clinicians' needs are met by conferences such as those analyzed.

Pickering (1984) used a qualitative rather than quantitative method to obtain a different perspective on interpersonal communication during supervision conferences, with evaluation procedures derived from phenomenology (Guba & Lincoln, 1981) and hermeneutics (Bender, 1975). She completed verbatim transcriptions of 40 10-to 15-minute audiotaped segments from the conferences between two supervisors and 10 student clinicians during one semester. The individual statements during conferences were first classified according to four a priori "sensitizing" concepts (sharing thoughts and feelings about self, being aware of others' thoughts and feelings, focusing on objective issues, and responding negatively to others) and three additional concepts that "emerged" during data analysis (students' interpersonal problems with clients, supervisors' instructional behaviors, and discussions about supervisor-student interactions). The categorized data were then studied for themes and patterns, upon which the author's conclusions were based. A consistency measure corresponding to reliability was obtained by having two colleagues categorize a sample of data according to the a priori sensitizing concepts. The categorizations were similar, with additional interpretations of interest to the study offered from the slightly different perspectives of the judges. A measure of truth value corresponding to internal validity was obtained by having the supervisors write in a journal following each conference to indicate similarity between their personal reflections about the conference and interpretations from the transcripts. The journal entries supported the findings from the transcripts and added important information of their own. Thus, both verification procedures provided primary data of interest as well as confirming the analyses of conference interactions.

Pickering's findings agreed closely with the findings of the quantitative research on supervision. Interpersonal communication during conferences was primarily instructional, with students reporting and supervisors advising. Discussion of interpersonal problems tended to concern students and clients rather than students and supervisors, with the students tending to attribute problems to the clients. The supervisors reinforced and supported the student, but did not explore the students' feelings or share their own feelings, even though the journal entries discussed feelings concerning interpersonal relationships with students. The conferences tented to be "helper-helpee" interactions rather than collaboration in joint problem solving. On the basis of these findings, the author concluded, like Roberts and Smith (1982), that the emphasis on instruction and technical skills rather than on self-evaluation and interpersonal skills in the conferences analyzed did not fit supervision models that call for self-exploration, interpersonal and intrapersonal growth, and collaborative problem solving (Anderson, 1981; Oratio, 1977). Pickering's qualitative study is important because it demonstrates the same general findings as quantitative studies by a different approach and provides additional insight about discrepancies between theoretical models of supervision and actual conference behavior.

Method of Supervison

Most supervision conferences appear to involve a discussion of the student clinician's progress in which the student supplies information about therapy in answer to the supervisor's questions, and the supervisor makes suggestions about strategy. Cimorell-Strong and Ensley (1982) introduced a variation by having one group of student clinicians give supervisors written feedback after each conference regarding their effectiveness in supervision. The students were beginning their first practicum and the supervisors had at least three years' experience. In one group of nine student–supervisor pairs, the students filled out a supervisor evaluation form (adapted from the Pennsylvania State University Evaluation Form) after six conferences within six weeks. A comparison group of seven student–supervisor pairs did not use evaluation forms. All conferences were audiotaped and a five-minute segment of each conference was analyzed by the method of Culatta and Seltzer (1976, 1977). The general pattern of interactions agreed with that reported by Culatta and Seltzer, with supervisor-dominated conferences and relatively infrequent evaluation, except that the present supervisors made more informational comments. The only differences between the two groups were that the supervisors in the no-feedback group made significantly more bad evaluations than those in the feedback group and that students in the feedback group asked more questions than the other students. In both groups the percentage of questions asked by supervisors decreased across the six-week period. The authors suggested that the public school supervisors used in their study made more information statements because they were more familiar with the students' clients than were the university supervisors in Culatta and Seltzer's studies and that the decrease in supervisors' questions reflected an increase in the students' skills.

Peaper (1984) introduced another variation in the study of supervisory conferences. She administered a 16-item questionnaire about the perceived value of the supervisory conference to graduate student clinicians at the beginning and end of a seven-week period in which 10 students prepared agendas for supervisory conferences and 11 students did not. The group as a whole rated conferences positively on both occasions. The only significant change over the seven-week period was an increase in the conviction of the students who prepared agendas that the students set the tone of the conference.

Dowling (1983a) studied the effect of a major variation in supervision method, a highly-structured teaching clinic. This approach, adapted from the field of education, involved a supervisor, a demonstration clinician, and other student clinicians. She analyzed five-minute segments of all parts of the teaching clinic during the students' second and fourth weeks. These clinics involved two teams of five students and one supervisor. The segments were analyzed by the Smith and Anderson (1982b) adaptation of the MOSAICS procedure. Other data included student ratings of the teaching clinic on a 16-item scale and interviews with the supervisors regarding their perceptions of the teaching clinic. The MOSAICS analyses indicated that most of the discussions involved supervisor-dominated questions and structuring, with discussions of methodology and objectives by students. There was minimal evaluation. The students rated the teaching clinic as increasing their clinical skills, but the majority would have liked more supervision. One supervisor thought that the teaching clinics forced students to become more involved, and the other supervisor believed that the clinic was valuable but did not provide enough guidance for beginning clinicians. The results would have been clearer if a less complex interactive analysis system than MOSAICS had been used. Dowling did not use the Culatta and Seltzer system because she and her colleagues (Dowling, Sbaschnig & Williams, 1982) had found the system to be neither reliable nor valid.

In a further study Dowling (1983b) compared the teaching clinic with conventional supervision conferences, using a counterbalanced procedure in which one team had four teaching clinics followed by four weeks of conventional supervision, and the other team had the same conditions in the opposite order. There were significant differences between conventional supervison and teaching clinics for five of 23 MOSAICS categories, but the results could not be clearly interpreted.

Pretraining of Clinical Skills

The amount and type of training in clinical skills prior to beginning supervised clinical training also has been studied. Volz, Klevans, Norton, and Putens (1978) wished to determine whether special training would improve the interpersonal skills of prepracticum students. In a post-training interview with a simulated client, they evaluated the interpersonal skills of 19 students who practiced individual helping skills, 15 students who used a role-playing method to learn helping skills, and a control group of 17 students who did not receive interpersonal skills training during an eight-week training period. The results were disappointing. None of the groups exhibited effective interpersonal skills, and the groups did not differ significantly, even when their interpersonal skills were assessed a second time during a practicum therapy session. The authors speculated that speech–language pathology students were not as well motivated to use interpersonal skills as students in counseling or social work, that training was insufficient compared to that given students in other disciplines, and that the initial level of interpersonal skills had not been controlled. They next assessed interpersonal skills during simulated helping interactions in 43 untrained prepracticum speech–language pathology students and 43 human service students enrolled in a course dealing with helping relationships. The interpersonal skills of the speech–language pathology students were found to be similar to the students trained in the previous study and were less effective than those of the human service students.

In a later study, Klevans, Volz, and Friedman (1981) attempted to develop effective short-term programs for training interpersonal skills, because there is not sufficient time available in the curriculum for long-term training programs. An Experiential group of 24 students was given seven training sessions that combined the helping skills and role playing methods used by Volz and colleagues (1978), and a Coding Practice group of 44 students was given seven sessions of training involving observation of role models and coding of clinical interactions. Except for a lower rate of open-ended questions, the responses of the Experiential group were interpreted as more effective than those of the Coding group in a post-training simulated helping interaction. Nevertheless, they used fewer facilitating responses than students in other disciplines who had had more training. It was noted that only six percent of the responses of the Experiential group reflected feelings, as compared with 49 percent of the responses of students in other disciplines. The results for the Coding group were similar to those of the prepracticum groups in the previous study. The authors concluded that more training is needed, and that speech–language pathology students do need to use interpersonal skills, particularly in the early stages of therapy.

Irwin (1981) compared two methods for teaching skills used in treating misarticulations. Both groups of prepracticum students began by studying a training manual and then completed three sessions of therapy training. A Model group of seven students viewed a videotaped demonstration of skills after the first and the second training sessions, and a Nonmodel group of eight students did not. Learning was evaluated by judging videotapes of the training sessions. Both groups improved significantly from the first to the second training session, with the Model group showing an almost significantly larger improvement than the Nonmodel group. (The difference probably would have been significant if a different method of statistical analysis had been used.) Individual differences in improvement indicated that some students required more training. The author speculated as to whether an efficiently designed technical skills training program might eliminate the need for "live" supervision.

SUMMARY OF RESEARCH TRENDS

Some useful practical findings emerged from the research reviewed here, with certain issues unresolved. Many of the findings regarding the characteristics of student clinicians were quite consistent. Supervisors, student clinicians, and clients shared the perception that professional–technical skills and interpersonal clinician–client skills are important components of clinical competence (Haynes & Oratio, 1978; Oratio, 1976a, 1978b; Shriberg et al., 1975, 1977). Clients attached little importance to the age, sex, race, or personal appearance of clinicians (Haynes & Oratio, 1978). Supervisors tended to grade students on the basis of technical skills (Shriberg et al., 1975), and the brightest, most stable students with the highest academic grades and the strongest interest in clinical work tended to receive the highest clinical grades (Shriberg et al., 1977). Technical skills were highly correlated with interpersonal skills (Oratio, 1978a;

Shriberg et al., 1975, 1977). Outstanding student clinicians tended to receive the highest supervisor ratings, and failing student clinicians received the lowest supervisor ratings on all clinical skills (Dowling, 1985), but good or poor student clinicians did not differ significantly on certain measures of cognitive–linguistic skill (Dowling & Bliss, 1984). Student clinicians as a group were not anxious about their clinical skills and tended to grow more confident as they gained experience (Sleight, 1985). Their confidence appeared justified, because their self-ratings of clinical skill tended to agree with those of their supervisors (Dowling, 1984) except for technical skills (Oratio, 1978b). Most student clinicians received good clinical grades (Dowling, 1985; Shriberg et al., 1977) and clinical skill ratings (Oratio, 1976a) from their supervisors.

The one area of confusion concerning the characteristics of student clinicians was the level of their interpersonal skills prior to beginning clinical training. Some evidence suggested that beginning student clinicians tended to have better interpersonal than technical skills (Oratio, 1978b; Shriberg et al., 1975). Other evidence indicated that prepracticum students had ineffective interpersonal skills in comparison with students in other helping professions and that lengthy training was required to bring the skills to an adequate level (Klevans et al., 1981; Volz et al., 1978).

Research on supervisors' characteristics did not yield as consistent a description as research on student clinicians' characteristics. Supervisors were expected to have a wide range of professional-technical and interpersonal skills (Oratio et al., 1981). In 1975, they described themselves as tending to have little supervision training or experience but feeling adequately prepared and supervising many students (Schubert & Aitchison, 1975). Research findings regarding their skills and attitudes were not flattering. Supervisors were found to be extremely inconsistent in rating student therapy sessions (Runyan & Seal, 1985) and strongly influenced by preconceptions about the students' clinical experience (Oratio, 1976b). They tended to hold the student completely responsible for the effectiveness of therapy (Roberts & Naremore, 1983). Nevertheless, they received very high ratings from student clinicians in all domains of competence (Oratio et al., 1981). When rating supervisor effectiveness, the student clinicians appeared to concentrate on supervisor–student interpersonal skills (Crichton & Oratio, 1984; Oratio et al., 1981). When rating their needs for supervision, beginning students wanted help in many aspects of supervision, and advanced students wanted to be relatively independent, but with different sets of needs stipulated by students in different training programs (Dowling & Wittkopp, 1982). Students ratings of supervisors did not appear to agree closely with the self-ratings of supervisors, whose overall opinion of their own effectiveness was lower than that of the students (Sleight, 1984).

Research on supervisor–student interactions during supervision conferences was consistent in indicating that conferences tended to be supervisor-dominated and analytic rather than student-centered and evaluative. Low-inference ratings suggested a stereotyped pattern of supervisor domination that did not change during clinical training despite supervisors' awareness of the pattern (Culatta & Seltzer, 1976, 1977). Nor did the pattern of supervisor domination change as a function of supervision method (Cimorell–Strong & Ensley, 1982; Dowling & Shank, 1981). However, the reliability and validity of the Culatta–Seltzer rating scale was questioned (Dowling, Sbaschnig & Williams, 1982). High-inference ratings indicated that the two most prominent modes of interaction were supervisor-dominated direct supervision and indirect supervision involving cooperative supervisor–student interactions (Brasseur & Anderson, 1983; Smith & Anderson, 1982a). When the high-inference ratings were made in conjunction with a complex low-inference system, the direct supervision mode was found to be associated with sequences of supervisor-dominated interactions, and the indirect supervision mode was associated with more student participation and discussion of feelings (Smith & Anderson, 1982b). Further analysis indicated that the supervisor-dominated mode was most frequent and did not change during clinical training (Roberts & Smith, 1982). Low-inference qualitative ratings also indicated that conferences were supervisor-dominated and instructional rather than evaluative, despite supervisors' private concerns about their feelings and those of the students (Pickering, 1984).

There has not been much systematic research on the effects of varying the methods used in the supervision conference. When students prepared an agenda for the conference, they experienced a greater sense of participation (Peaper, 1984). In addition, when they gave written feedback to supervisors following conferences, the supervisors made fewer negative evaluations and the students asked more questions (Cimorell-Strong & Ensley, 1982). A structured teaching clinic involving student peers appeared to be just as dominated by the supervisor as conventional conferences when analyzed by the complex low-inference rating system, but with some differences that could not be interpreted (Dowling, 1983a,b).

The extent to which clinical skills can be taught prior to supervised practicum training has also been investigated. Human Communication Disorders students were found to have ineffective interpersonal skills relevant to therapy interactions, and these skills were not easily taught (Klevans et al., 1981; Volz et al., 1978). Nevertheless, there was some indication that specific technical skills could be taught prior to practicum training (Irwin, 1981).

EVALUATION OF RESEARCH

Researchers have shown a great deal of ingenuity in conceptualizing and devising appropriate methods of investigating important issues concerning supervision. Notable are the variety of studies by Dowling and Oratio and their coworkers and the rigorous analyses of supervision conference interactions by Anderson and Smith and their collaborators. The substantial investigations of Shriberg and his collaborators and of Klevans and Volz and their colleagues represent communication disorders research at its best. Pickering's qualitative research is an indispensable antidote to the otherwise uniformly quantitative approaches to supervision research. These investigators have opened up many paths for further research.

Researchers have concentrated on the competence of student clinicians and supervisors and on student–supervisor interactions during supervision conferences. They have not yet come to grips with the basic issues of how supervision contributes to the eventual competence of the practicing clinician and how supervision might be improved through supervisor selection and training and new methods of supervision. There seems to be agreement about theoretical models of the multiskilled student clinician and supervisor and a common opinion that the goals of supervision conferences should extend beyond the perfection of technical and interpersonal clinician–client skills to the fostering of joint personal growth through empathic interactions of students and supervisors.

Methodology is a matter of active concern, as it should be. Subjective ratings, mail questionnaires, and correlational studies have well-known pitfalls. The use of subjective ratings for supervision research seems appropriate, because supervisors' ratings of students and students' self-ratings are used in clinical training. Nevertheless, the findings that supervisors' ratings may be overuniform in some respects and inconsistent and biased in other respects and that students' ratings are influenced by their training program suggest that other ways of assessing clinical competence and supervisor competence must be found.

Mail questionnaires have contributed useful information, because they sample a wide range of training programs. Nevertheless, a systematic bias may be introduced by the lack of information about those who fail to return the questionnaires. The findings of questionnaire studies should be corroborated by procedures that avoid self-selection bias.

Correlational studies demonstrate relationships among numerical measures but do not necessarily reveal the structure of the underlying abilities. Where the numerical measures are subjective ratings, inferences become more tenuous. Factor analysis, which is based upon intercorrelations, can provide a parsimonious description of a large number of measures by grouping highly correlated measures into factors. However, measures that are not classified into factors should not be discarded as meaningless. For example, in the factor analysis of student-rated supervisor skills (Oratio et al., 1981), 38 of the 45 items were not classified into any factors, and the factor structure should have been interpreted as indeterminate rather than "a parsimonious two-factor solution" (p. 39). There should be further investigation into the structure of supervision skills.

Technology may also pose a problem in interpreting some studies. Audiotapes may yield different information than videotapes concerning certain supervision conference interactions.

RECOMMENDATIONS FOR FURTHER RESEARCH

A number of suggestions regarding further research have already been made. Simple but valid and reliable low-inference conference rating systems are needed. Because the Culatta-Seltzer system seems useful, perhaps it could be made more valid and reliable. Alternatives to subjective ratings should be found for research on clinical and supervisor competence and on supervision conference interactions. The use of qualitative methodology by Pickering provides at least one promising alternative, but qualitative methods have their own problems — notably the amount of time required for data reduction and analysis and the extent to which the results from small samples of supervisors and students can be generalized. Changes in clinical competence as a result of supervision should be studied in relation to the eventual competence of practicing clinicians. The effects of super visor training should be determined, as should the effects of variations in supervision methods.

If possible, individual difference variables such as age, sex, cultural background, and training of students and supervisors should be varied systematically, as should the types of assessment and treatment involved in clinical training. The majority of research has dealt with speech–language pathology supervision in general, which could be subdivided into different childhood and adult disorders. Supervision in audiology and in education of hearing-impaired children should also be studied. Comparisons with supervision in related disciplines might also be informative. Finally, the effects of new methods of computerized assessment and treatment on supervised clinical training should be studied.

CONCLUSIONS

Supervision research is a healthy enterprise that will continue to provide useful information. What conclusions might we draw on the basis of research to date? Almost all students receive good grades from their supervisors. Is this because clinical training is more effective than academic training, students have more aptitude for clinical than for academic skills, or supervisors are too lenient in judging clinical skills? How can we put together research that finds that supervisors are inconsistent, biased, and unsure of themselves; confident and satisfied with themselves; domineering, analytic, and non-evaluative in supervision conferences; and privately concerned with their own feelings and those of the students? A large proportion of graduates in Human Communication Disorders are pressed into service as supervisors after only one or two years of practice and with little or no training in supervision, and have to work with many students. Perhaps they have little alternative but to use the time available in supervision conferences to advise the student on technical and interpersonal skills rather than engaging in open-ended student-centered discussions. Researchers should continue to look for better ways to find out more about the thoughts, feelings, and interactions of supervisors and those they supervise, many of whom will themselves become supervisors.

REFERENCES

Anderson, J. L. (1981). Training of supervisors in speech–language pathology and audiology. *Asha, 23,* 77–82.

Aram, D. M. & Nation, J. E. (1975). Patterns of language behavior in children with developmental language disorders. *Journal of Speech and Hearing Research, 18,* 229–241.

Bender, H. E. (1975). Dilthey's voice in the emerging consciousness of humanistic education. *Journal of Education,* (Boston University), *157*(1), 31–34.

Boone, D. R. & Prescott, T. E. (1972). Content and sequence analysis of speech and hearing therapy. *Asha, 14,* 58–62.

Brasseur, J. A. & Anderson, J. L. (1983). Observed differences between direct, indirect, and direct/indirect videotaped supervisory conferences. *Journal of Speech and Hearing Research, 26,* 349–355.

Caracciolo, G. L. (1977). Perceptions by speech pathology student clinicians and supervisors of interpersonal conditions and professional growth during the supervisory conference. *Dissertation Abstracts International, 37,* 4411B. (University Microfilms No. 77-04, 183).

Cimorell-Strong, J. M. & Ensley, K. G. (1982). Effects of student clinician feedback on the supervisory conference. *Asha, 24,* 23–29.

Crichton, L. J. & Oratio, A. R. (1984). Speech–language pathologists' clinical fellowship training. Asha, 26, 39–43.

Culatta, R., Colucci, S. & Wiggins, E. (1975). Clinical supervisors and trainees: Two views of a process. *Asha, 17,* 152–157.

Culatta, R. & Seltzer, H. (1976). Content and sequence analysis of the supervisory session. *Asha, 18,* 8–12.

Culatta, R. & Seltzer, H. (1977). Content and sequence analysis of the supervisory session: A report of clinical use. *Asha, 19,* 523–526.

Dowling, S. (1983a). Teaching clinic conference participant interaction. *Journal of Communication Disorders, 16,* 385–397.

Dowling, S. (1983b). An analysis of conventional and teaching clinic supervision. *The Clinical Supervisor, 1*(4), 15–29.

Dowling, S. (1984). Clinical evaluation: A comparison of self, self with videotape, peers, and supervisors. *The Clinical Supervisor, 2*(3), 71–78.

Dowling, S. (1985). Clinical performance characteristics: Failing, average, and outstanding clinicians. *The Clinical Supervisor, 3*(3), 49–54.

Dowling, S. & Bliss, L. S. (1984). Cognitive complexity, rhetorical sensitivity: Contributing factors in clinical skill? *Journal of Communication Disorders, 17,* 9–17.

Dowling, S., Sbaschnig, K. V. & Williams, C. J. (1982). Culatta and Seltzer content and sequence analysis of the supervisory session: Question of reliability and validity. *Journal of Communication Disorders, 15,* 353–362.

Dowling, S. & Shank, K. H. (1981). A comparison of the effects of two supervisory styles, conventional and teaching clinic, in the training of speech and language pathologists. *Journal of Communication Disorders, 14,* 51–58.

Dowling, S. & Wittkopp, J. (1982). Students' perceived supervisory needs. *Journal of Communication Disorders, 15,* 319–328.

Guba, E. G. & Lincoln, Y. S. (1981). *Effective evaluation.* San Francisco: Jossey-Bass.

Haynes, W. O. & Oratio, A. R. (1978). A study of clients' perceptions of therapeutic effectiveness. *Journal of Speech and Hearing Disorders, 43,* 21–33.

Klevans, D. R., Volz, H. B. & Friedman, R. M. (1981). A comparison of experiential and observational approaches for enhancing the interpersonal communication skills of speech–language pathology students. *Journal of Speech and Hearing Disorders, 46,* 208–213.

Irwin, R. B. (1975). Microcounseling interviewing skills of supervisors of speech clinicians. *Human Communication, 4,* 5–9.

Irwin, R. B. (1981). Training speech pathologists through microtherapy. *Journal of Communication Disorders, 14,* 93–103.

Oratio, A. R. (1976a). A factor analytic study of criteria for evaluating student clinicians in speech pathology. *Journal of Communication Disorders, 9,* 199–210.

Oratio, A. R. (1976b). The clinician's level of training as a factor in supervisors' evaluation of clinical performance. *Ohio Journal of Speech and Hearing, 12,* 21–35.

Oratio, A. R. (1977). *Supervison in speech pathology: A handbook for supervisors and clinicians.* Baltimore, MD: University Park Press.

Oratio, A. R. (1978a). Interrelationship between interpersonal and technical skills of student clinicians in speech therapy. *Acta Symbolica, 7,* 29–41.

Oratio, A. R. (1978b). Comparative perceptions of therapeutic effectiveness by student clinicians and clinical supervisors. *Asha, 20,* 959–962.

Oratio, A. R. (1980). Dimensions of therapeutic behavior. *Journal of Communication Disorders, 13,* 213–230.

Oratio, A. R., Sugarman, M. & Prass, M. (1981). A multivariate analysis of clinicians' perceptions of supervisory effectiveness. *Journal of Communication Disorders, 14,* 31–42.

Peaper, R. E. (1984). An analysis of student perceptions of the supervisory conference and student-developed agendas for that conference. *The Clinical Supervisor, 2*(1), 55–69.

Pickering, M. (1984). Interpersonal communication in speech–language pathology supervisory conference: A qualitative study. *Journal of Speech and Hearing Disorders, 49,* 189–195.

Roberts, J. E. & Naremore, R. C. (1983). An attributional model of supervisors' decision-making behavior in speech–language pathology. *Journal of Speech and Hearing Research, 26,* 537–549.

Roberts, J. E. & Smith, K. J. (1982). Supervisor–supervisee role differences and consistency of behavior in supervisory conferences. *Journal of Speech and Hearing Research, 25,* 428–434.

Runyan, S. E. & Seal, B. C. (1985). A comparison of supervisors' ratings while observing a language remediation session. *The Clinical Supervisor, 3,* 61–75.

Schubert, G. W. & Aitchison, C. J. (1975). A profile of clinical supervisors in college and university speech and hearing training programs. *Asha, 17,* 440–447.

Shriberg, L. D., Bless, D. M., Carlson, K. A., Filley, F. S., Kwiatkowski, J. & Smith, M. E. (1977). Personality characteristics, academic performance, and clinical competence in communicative disorders majors. *Asha, 19,* 311–321.

Shriberg, L. D., Filley, F. S., Hayes, D. M. Kwiatkowski, J, Schatz, J. A., Simmons, K. M. & Smith, M. E. (1975). The Wisconsin Procedure for

Appraisal of Clinical Competence (W-PACC): Model and data. *Asha, 17,* 158–165.

Sleight, C. C. (1984). Supervisor self-evaluation in communication disorders. *The Clinical Supervisor, 2*(3), 31–42.

Sleight, C. C. (1985). Confidence and anxiety in student clinicians. *The Clinical Supervisor, 3*(3), 25–47.

Smith, K. J. & Anderson, J. L. (1982a). Development and validation of an individual supervisory conference rating scale for use in speech-pathology. *Journal of Speech and Hearing Research, 25,* 243–251.

Smith, K. J. & Anderson, J. L. (1982b). Relationship of perceived effectiveness to verbal interaction/content variables in supervisory conferences in speech–language pathology. *Journal of Speech and Hearing Research, 25,* 252–261.

Ulrich, S. R. & Watt, J. (1977, November). Competence of clinical supervisors: A statistical analysis. Annual meeting of the American Speech, Language and Hearing Association. Chicago, IL.

Volz, H. B., Klevans, D. R., Norton, S. J. & Putens, D. L. (1978). Interpersonal communication skills of speech–language pathology undergraduates: The effects of training. *Journal of Speech and Hearing Disorders, 43,* 524–542.

Weller, R. H. (1971). *Verbal communication in instructional supervision.* New York: Teachers College Press.

CHAPTER 5

Supervision:
A Person-Focused Process

Marisue Pickering

S upervision in the field of Human Communication Disorders is a person-focused process. Human interaction is its primary context, focus, and tool. Scholars in supervision have examined important, person-focused aspects of the supervisory experience and process, including conference interactions (e.g., Roberts & Smith, 1982; Smith & Anderson, 1982), supervisory styles (e.g., Brasseur & Anderson, 1983), students' perceptions (e.g., Dowling & Wittkopp, 1982; Wollman & Conover, 1979), and interpersonal skill training (e.g., Volz, Klevans, Norton & Putens, 1978). Furthermore, supervisors have used the person-focused humanistic perspective to define and describe what this dynamic, human process is or could be about (e.g., Oratio, 1977; Pickering, 1977). Models for structuring supervision as an *interactive* process have been suggested (e.g., Anderson, 1981; Oratio, 1977), and people-oriented, professional issues have been identified (e.g., Gavett, 1985; Kennedy, 1985; Pickering, 1985; Rassi, 1985). There exist, however, numerous other features and nuances of a person-focused process that have yet to be discussed. The purpose of this chapter is to initiate such a discussion.

The chapter begins by contextualizing supervision as being person-focused. Parallels between the clinical and supervisory processes in Human Communication Disorders are identified, and an analogous relationship between the two processes is suggested. In the second section, epistemological considerations, that is, paradigms used for knowing and understanding reality, are briefly discussed. In addition, approaches to knowing and understanding reality within the field of Human Communication Disorders are identified. The next section considers three major constructs that are integral to one particular approach to understanding — the interpretive-phenomenological approach as explicated in the human sciences. The discussion also relates these constructs — interpretation, accounts of human action, and linguistic expression — to supervision. The chapter's conclusion takes the form of a set of implications and assertions that arise out of the prior discussion.

SUPERVISION AS A PERSON-FOCUSED PROCESS

Supervision means being person-focused. To begin with, the participants in the working relationship (supervision) and in the highlighted relationship (therapy) are people; the two sets of relationships are, by definition, interpersonal; and the medium for and outcome of both student learning and client change is human communication.

Supervision is person-focused because it is concerned with human growth and change, not only for clients, but also for students. The term *growth,* although not operationally defined, is found often in the supervisory literature. From its earliest writings, this literature has contained a sub-theme and, at times, a primary theme concerned with growth of the student–clinician, a growth that goes beyond, but perhaps is the base for, the acquisition and improvement of specified technical skills of intervention and diagnosis, as well as improved interpersonal and counseling skills. Ward and Webster (1965) spoke about providing conditions for students' self-actualization as well as experiences through which they could explore and exercise "their own humanness" (p. 39). These authors argued for the application of person-focused clinical concepts to the training and preparation of students. They questioned whether students could provide conditions for the growth of their clients if the same were not being done for them. Pickering (1984) has raised the issue of the purpose of the supervisory conference relative to both interpersonal and intrapersonal growth. She noted that if personal growth is valued by supervisors, aspects of the conference interaction will need to be structured to that end.

Supervision is person-focused in that within the process, students are expected to merge who they are personally with whom they are becoming professionally. Oratio (1977), for example, discussed helping students self-explore their "clinical personality" and suggested this be a fundamental purpose of the conference interaction (p. 134). Furthermore, his work suggests the importance of students engaging in "deep clinical self-exploration" vis-à-vis the therapeutic encounter (p. 106). Caracciolo, Rigrodsky, and Morrison (1978) were also concerned about this aspect of clinical training. They discussed the need for student–clinicians to be able to express "opinions, attitudes, and knowledge with respect to the client" (p. 288) and suggested a particular supervisory orientation (based on the work of psychotherapist Carl Rogers) that could facilitate such expresssion.

Supervision is person-focused in that supervisors examine aspects of themselves — something they were called on to do by Ward and Webster (1965), who stated "we must clarify our views of ourselves as teachers, supervisors, and members of a clinical profession" (p. 40). Such clarification can take many forms. For example, Anderson's (1981) model of supervision assumes the necessity of supervisors' using self-analysis techniques. Pickering and McCready (1983), using findings from supervisory journal analysis, reported supervisors' explorations of their own personal growth and meanings vis-à-vis encounters with students. McCrea (1980) looked at supervisors' use of the facilitative dimensions of concreteness, genuineness, respect, and empathic understanding within conferences, and Ellis (1986) reported an approach to supervisory self-confrontation based on conference tape analysis. Within this book, Crago (chap. 6) discusses supervisors' use of self-exploration as a tool for enhancing supervisory skills, and McCready, Shapiro, and Kennedy (chap. 7) suggest inter- and intrapersonal dynamics that may influence supervisors. Self-examination of a different type includes Gavett (1985), Kennedy (1985), Pickering (1985), and Rassi's (1985) discussions of supervisors' personal and professional concerns and related issues vis-à-vis academic institutions. These writers examined issues more concerned with being a supervisor than with the supervisory process per se.

Supervision is person-focused because it is interactive in nature, which means that there exists an infinite number and variety of human behaviors that can be attended to, or ignored. There exist dimensions, subtleties, and nuances of human interaction to be responded to, or ignored. There exists a constant set of professional, communicative, moral, and ethical options from which to choose when interacting. The interactive dimensions of this process reflect the fact that supervision, like other person-focused processes, is a complex phenomenon. Without making supervision into a mystique, it is valid to assert that "in order for clinical supervision to be understood by those who don't do it, the person-focus of both the process and of the supervisors, themselves, must be understood" (Pickering, 1985, p. 18).

The Clinical Process and the Supervisory Process

Given that supervision is carried out by people who are certified as clinicians and that it developed in order to help students become clinicians, it is to be expected that aspects of the clinical process would be seen as applicable to the supervisory process. For example, Ward and Webster (1965) stated, "We must apply clinically valid concepts about human beings to students as well as to clinic clients" (p. 40). Moreover, Van Riper (1965) noted that "To be a clinician you must care. We have found it important to show some of that same interest and concern for the students we supervise" (p. 77). For Murphy (1982), the supervisory relationship is akin to the clinical relationship: "The relationship between the speech–language pathologist and the supervisor is . . . in many respects, representative of what happens in the clinician–client relationship" (p. 458).

Certain areas of correspondence between the two relationships and processes are quite clear. In the clinical literature, the importance of human development, of growth, and of the interpersonal relationship has been an ongoing theme (e.g., Cooper, et al., 1982; Emerick & Hood, 1974; Travis, 1957). As noted earlier, this theme has also been present in the supervision literature. Perhaps its presence in the writings about both processes can be explained by suggesting that it is a value strongly held by the discipline and explicitly articulated by particular clinicians and supervisors. Some of the writers who discuss human growth and the importance of relationships clearly have been influenced by the intellectual traditions of existential philosophy, phenomenology, or humanistic psychology (Caracciolo, Rigrodsky & Morrison, 1978; Gildston & Gildston, 1972; Martin, 1963; Murphy, 1982; Oratio, 1977; Pickering, 1977). Perhaps other writers are reflecting traditional helping attitudes such as those articulated by Brammer (1985) in his work on the process and skills of helping relationships.

Whatever the grounding or the influences, doing therapy and doing supervision correspond along the dimension of valuing human growth and the interpersonal relationship.

Human Communication Disorders is a helping field; the clinical relationship is a helping relationship. Similarly, the supervisory relationship can be viewed as a helping relationship, an idea suggested by Caracciolo, Rigrodksy, and Morrison (1978). Thus, the supervisory relationship would have meaning and structure for its participants beyond being simply a context for teaching or learning clinical skills. What the meaning is for its participants remains an open issue — as it does in the clinical process. Although there has not been much discussion in the literature of clients' views of clinical relationships, when there has been such a discussion (e.g., Chubrich, 1978), the profession is reminded of what the experience signifies for a client. In supervision, there is even less literature on the meaning of either the process or the relationship for its participants. One report comes from Pickering (1981), who quoted a university supervisor as stating, "To me, growth is the ultimate goal as well as an ongoing process in the supervisory interaction — growth of client, of clinician, and of supervisor." Pickering also quoted a student who stated:

> I have definitely felt a challenge to grow as a person in order to meet certain clinical expectations. I feel that I have developed more in the area of disciplining myself. Also, I have learned much more about what commitment and responsibility mean. This has all been very positive for me — a very good lesson. (p. 21)

Even on this little evidence, it can be assumed that the supervisory relationship is significant to both participants beyond teaching or learning specified skills.

Another area of correspondence between the clinical and supervisory processes concerns their structure. Both processes have a particular structure, or "anatomy," a term used by Thomas (1984, part II) in his discussion of helping professions. A component within the structure of each process is that one person is identified as the *helper* and the other as the *helpee*. In both processes, the helpee is expected to meet certain identifiable objectives through a process of change. In the clinical process, these objectives are usually specified as goals and subgoals (e.g., see Fey, 1986; Hess, 1976). In the supervisory process, the objectives for the helpee (the student) may be stated as skills to be evaluated (e.g., Shriberg, et al., 1975) or as competencies to be achieved (e.g., Johnson, Prudhomme & Rogero, 1982).

The two processes share other features, and it is likely that supervisors have brought from the clinical experience knowledge of how to order and work with these features. Such features, which are associated with helping professions in general (Thomas, 1984), include introducing, reinforcing, and shaping new behaviors. Both processes also allow for monitoring, evaluating, and giving feedback about change. And, of course, both processes structure opportunities for generalization. In addition, moral and ethical choices are present in both processes, as they are in helping professions in general (Thomas, 1984). For example, moral considerations apply if the helper evokes in clients or students anxieties and fears that they do not have the necessary skills to handle, or if they are pushed toward change in ways that leave them bewildered or with significantly lowered self-esteem. In addition, ethical considerations are present when a client or student shows little or no progress within the parameters of the helping process.

Another area of correspondence concerns the use of theoretical models. Both processes are concerned with models for intervention per se as well as with models of the structure of the process. Model development probably comes about because of the practitioner's need to make sense of, order, refine, articulate, and teach the process being experienced. Models underpinning clinical work are numerous and familiar and are often summarized in clinical texts, for example, by Fey (1986) in children's language disorders and by Ham (1986) in stuttering therapy.

In supervision, Oratio (1977) developed the "Molar Model," which provides a framework for achieving goals specific to a clinician's development. This model identifies specific elements of the supervisory process, such as observation, conferences, and live demonstration. Its basic method is study and analysis of the student's therapeutic behavior (p. 138). Anderson (1981) also developed a model of supervision, one in which both supervisor and supervisee share problem-solving related to client or program needs (p. 79). This model, based on the Clinical Supervision Model developed in education by Cogan (1973) and Goldhammer (1969), includes the use of self-analysis techniques by supervisors and students and stresses the collection of data. The interaction between supervisor and student is viewed as important as well as measurable. Other models developed for the supervisory process include one based on a Rogerian orientation (Caracciolo, Rigrodsky & Morrison, 1978), one that is organized by stages with concomitant skill categories (Andreani & Peters, 1977), and one that is organized by levels of career training (Schoenberg, Larson & Gevaart, 1980–1981).

A final area of similarity between the two processes concerns those humanistic qualities or abilities that Gavett (1985) identified as "the ability to empathize, to inspire, to motivate, to listen, and to be non-judgmental" (p. 21). She identified these qualities as reflecting the "art" of supervision as compared and contrasted to the "science" of supervision. In a field that Perkins (1971) referred to as an applied behavioral science, viewing aspects of the clinical and supervisory processes as art may seem archaic. Nevertheless, there are feelings of appreciation and caring for the other person that have no single operational definition, areas of knowledge about what to do and say that are hard to translate into a competency, and important clinical and supervisory attitudes and intentions that are difficult to specify as skills. One such intention involves listening with an understanding that is based in human concern (Murphy, 1982, p. 468). This intention relates to Cole and Lacefield's (1978) skill domain of "showing and maintaining respect and regard for others, especially one's clients" (p. 117). Cole and Lacefield, authors who are concerned with the helping professions, consider such an attitude and its related behaviors critical.

As helping processes, both clinical work and supervision are open to influence and the application of criteria from the literature in the helping professions. Applying such criteria to both processes would explicate additional correspondences, and differences, in the two processes. For example, application of Cole and Lacefield's (1978) set of "skill domains" integral to helping professions could help reveal the analogous relationship of the two processes.

Seeing the parallels between the clinical and supervisory processes is not a difficult endeavor, nor is contextualizing the supervisory process as a person-focused process. The challenges come in efforts to understand subtleties and person-focused paradigms and theories, and then to apply the new knowledge within the supervisory process. In the next section, some ideas about ways of understanding reality or knowing the world are introduced and these ideas are then discussed in relation to the field in general and supervision in particular.

EPISTEMOLOGICAL CONSIDERATIONS

This introduction to epistemological considerations points out that different ways exist for knowing and understanding reality and implies that attention to a discipline's ways of knowing is critical.

Concern about the nature of knowing — epistemology — is an ancient one that often gets re-examined. Scholars have pondered both the basic assumptions out of which questions are asked and the operating paradigms out of which interpretations are made. Modern scholars such as Capra (from that parent of sciences, physics), Berman (from the history of science), and Polkinghorne (from the human sciences) are among those who have discussed general frameworks that structure approaches to knowing (Berman, 1981; Capra, 1982; Polkinghorne, 1983). Two frameworks emerge as providing differing ways through which to construct and then interpret and understand the world.

The first framework represents a logical positivist approach to knowing and is the more orthodox one (Polkinghorne, 1983). It depends on sense-data as a foundation for scientific research and seeks objective facts, usually through hypothesis testing and prediction. Berman (1981) discussed such a view of reality as being based on experiment, quantification, prediction, control, and technical mastery. Capra (1982) discussed the development of this framework as a particular worldview and linked it with the development of Newtonian physics. Both Berman and Capra believe that much of modern Western consciousness is rooted in this worldview, which is primarily mechanistic and deterministic.

A quite different way of knowing represents the tradition of the *human sciences,* a tradition that dates at least to Dilthey, a German philosopher of the late 19th century (Polkinghorne, 1983). Dilthey argued that the methodology of the human sciences must be different from the methodology of the natural sciences (Bender, 1975; Polkinghorne, 1983). The human sciences depend on experience as a foundation for scientific research and seek increased understanding of human experience. Thus, the foundation of the human sciences — experience — is that which is studied and which is also the tool of study (not unlike supervision). The human sciences call for a dialectical approach to understanding (Berger & Luckman, 1966; Berman, 1981; Darroch & Silvers, 1982), which acknowledges that individuals and their social worlds interact with each other. A dialectical approach also avows that knowledge is a factor in inquiry as well as its product. That is, what is known affects as well as effects what will be known. The human sciences thus acknowledge the inseparability of fact and value (Berman, 1981). The approaches to inquiry in the human science tradition are often descriptive, interpretive, existential and phenomenological and "are aimed at describing and clarifying the nature of experience which people live through" (Polkinghorne, 1983, p. 239).

Modern scholars in a variety of fields have been concerned about and have grappled with ways and kinds of knowing. For example, psychologist Abraham Maslow (1966) divided knowledge into spectator knowledge and experiential knowledge and suggested that in experiential knowledge, the observer is really a participant. Maslow stressed integrating the two approaches rather than dichotomizing them. He argued that "The two kinds of knowledge are necessary to each other and under good circumstances can be and should be intimately integrated with each other" (p. 49).

Child psychiatrist Robert Coles (1979), in his discussion of teaching medical ethics, probed two philosophical traditions he called the analytic and the existential. Coles noted that the analytic tradition allows for considering numerous variables and making specific medical decisions. The existential tradition allows for pondering the unique nature of each person as well as the particularities of daily life. In Coles' own prolific writings about, among other phenomena, the lives of children living in troublesome circumstances, he clearly is interested in the existential dimensions. Coles also views the existential dimension as important when considering how to teach ethics in medical schools.

Communication scholar Raymie McKerrow (1980) represents another field — rhetoric — that considers ways of knowing. In discussing the use of validation systems for the appraisal of arguments, McKerrow noted that many systems set up objectifiable standards that are based on the assumption that the arguments are seeking *truth*. Such an approach assumes the existence of truth. McKerrow noted that another set of standards may be needed in order to understand the nature of the relationship of the individuals involved. If the rhetorical discourse has as its intent and effect maintaining the relationship, applying a standard of validity that fails to take this intent and effect into account will preclude understanding what is happening. McKerrow identified the need for a second set of standards that would reflect a phenomenological perspective on argument discourse.

Another example of scholars concerned with ways and kinds of knowing comes from the work of Lakoff and Johnson (1980), scholars in linguistics and philosophy, respectively. These writers probed systems of knowing based on objectivism and its converse, subjectivism, and offered a third choice: an "experientialist synthesis" (p. 192). Lakoff and Johnson suggested that to be objective means believing in an objective reality, being rational, and assuming that reality can be described correctly. They suggested that being subjective means relying on intuitions, being emotional, and assuming that poetic expressions transcend rationality. They noted that objectivism allies with scientific truth and impartiality, and subjectivism with art and imagination. They argued that both objectivism and subjectivism are myths that miss the fact that individuals have a dialectical relationship with the world; that is, the world is understood through interacting with it in an ongoing way.

In addition to individual scholars trying to understand different ways of knowing, whole fields of inquiry are redefining their epistemologies as well as redefining what is known. Modern physics is an example of the former, and feminist theory is an example of the latter. Both are contributing to and are reflective of a major paradigm shift in both how to know and what to know. Moreover, both areas of inquiry are developing a new hermeneutics — interpretive rules — in an effort to understand the world in different ways.

Berman (1981), Capra (1982), and Wolf (1981) are among those writers who have noted that a paradigm shift is occurring in physics. The Newtonian worldview is being replaced by a view that understands phenomena in truly different ways. This new worldview has emerged from quantum mechanics. Among the implications of quantum mechanics for the concerns of supervision are (1) there is no such thing as an uninvolved observer, (2) knowledge about nature is indeterminate, and (3) phenomena (particles) have no meaning as isolated entities but can be understood only as part of a system (Berman, 1981; Capra, 1982; Wolf, 1981). The implications of a paradigm shift concerning the nature of knowing in physics have significant import, because so much of modern consciousness appears to have been influenced by the Newtonian worldview that posited a predictable, objective, and mechanistic view of the universe (Capra, 1982).

Another worldview is changing — that of androcentrism. A woman-centered perspective, feminist theory, and feminist hermeneutics are providing opportunities to see the world differently, from Biblical interpretations (Ruether, 1975) to parenting (Rich, 1976), from historical analysis (Lerner, 1979) to everyday language (Spender, 1980; Thorne, Kramarae & Henley, 1983). Among the implications of feminist theory for the concerns of supervision are (1) the importance of shared, collaborative decision-making; (2) the critique and demystification of power; (3) the importance of intimacy and nurturance; and (4) the use of multiple perspectives in viewing and understanding the world (Donovan, 1985; Eisenstein, 1983). Because so much of reality has been influenced by a male-centered perspective (Eisenstein, 1981; Ruether, 1975), a paradigm shift that provides for understanding experience from a perspective other than one that is male-centered is resulting in interpretations significantly different from traditional ones. Interestingly, some writers have postulated congruencies between modern feminist thought and modern physics (Donovan, 1985; Morgan, 1984).

All fields adhere to particular paradigms for knowing or understanding the reality of interest. In the next section, approaches to knowing in the field of Human Communication Disorders are considered.

Approaches to Knowing in Human Communication Disorders

The literature in Human Communication Disorders reflects the sense that the predominant paradigm in this field is based on a logical positivist way of knowing. Apparently this paradigm is taken for granted much of the time, especially in the research literature. For example, Silverman's (1985) work on research design includes no discussions of interpretive–phenomenological research or of the human sciences. Similarly, Shearer (1982) limited his discussion of research processes in speech, language, and hearing to traditional ones that he equated with the scientific method. As helpful as these books are, they do not consider any way of knowing other than a traditional one, nor do the writers acknowledge their own epistemological choice.

The question of being scientific (in the traditional sense) is tacitly or explicitly part of the clinical literature. Occasionally there is a concern with being *more* scientific; again the term *scientific* has a traditional connotation. Kamhi (1984), for example, discussed why clinical practice is not scientific and argued the need for clinicians to become clinical scientists. Without disclaiming the importance of Kamhi's argument, it can be noted, however, that the epistemological stance undergirding his argument is that there is one appropriate way for understanding and working with clinical reality and that way is based on the traditional scientific model.

Nevertheless, writers in Human Communication Disorders have suggested that there is more than one approach to knowing. Several examples are illustrative.

One exemplar is found in Gildston and Gildston's (1972) discussion of the contrast between existentialism and determinism, as ways of approaching intervention. These writers summarized these contrastive ways of knowing and illustrated the existential approach to working with aphasic, laryngectomized, and hard-of-hearing patients. In one of their case examples, they applied the existential principle of being involved with a patient's problems in the existential, present moment. The clinician no longer was the outside helper, but a member of the man's world, interacting with him and his family spontaneously and at an affective level. The clinician was not administering an intervention *to* a patient, but interacting *with* him and his family. For a brief time, the clinician had joined the family's world (p. 35).

Murphy (1974) discussed two ways of knowing when he considered the phenomenon of stuttering. He explicated an approach to understanding stuttering that calls for objective description, quantitative analysis, and a rational construction of the phenomenon. In addition, he discussed an approach that calls for the ability to empathize with the stuttering client; to understand what this person feels, thinks, fears, and hopes; and to conceive of stuttering through poetic imagery. In his delineation of these two approaches, Murphy articulated two ways of knowing the reality of stuttering and the world of the stuttering person, as well as two ways of approaching therapy.

In another discussion, Murphy (1985) delineated between traditional and nontraditional ways of considering research in special education. The traditional approach he saw as scientific, experimental, and quantitative. He considered nontraditional approaches to be phenomenological, existential, and qualitative. Murphy indicated that phenomenological perspectives are more difficult to find in professional journals than are traditional perspectives. Although Murphy identified the importance of both approaches, he noted that precisely defined abstractions, such as those found in traditional approaches, carry the risk of losing some of the richness of the phenomena being studied.

Another example comes from Siegel and Spradlin (1985) who developed the thesis that therapy and research differ along several dimensions. Although these writers did not focus their discussion on the paradigms undergirding therapy or research, they did argue that the goals and tactics for the two differ. Whether these authors see these two endeavors as operating out of different paradigms for understanding is unclear, in part because neither construct is explicated or defined. Furthermore, part of the essay discusses using the scientific method to guide therapy, but other parts clearly stress the importance of experiential knowledge in planning and providing intervention. It is not clear whether the scientific method is understood in inclusive or exclusive ways. Regardless of the way the authors themselves view the nature of knowing within therapy and research, their discussion raises the issue for the reader. Such an issue is an epistemological one.

A final exemplar is found in the work of Prutting (1983), in which she discussed aspects of both the hermeneutic and positivistic philosophies of science and made applications to Human Communication Disorders. It is clear that for Prutting, "scientific inquiry" and the field of science includes *both* philosophies. It is equally clear that Prutting believes that both philosophies (epistemologies) provide a basis from which to function in the discipline. Prutting's discussion includes a focus on the scientific parameters of objectivity/subjectivity, and she probes the modern myth that science is objective. On the issue of subjectivity, Prutting states, "One needs to realize that what one believes determines what questions to ask and how to ask them" (p. 253).

Prutting pointed out that the word *science* is rooted in the Latin *scientia,* meaning to know. Her essay noted that there are different ways of knowing, differing philosophies of science. Although Prutting did not use the term *human science,* her understanding of the hermeneutic tradition fits well with Polkinghorne's (1983) discussion of the human sciences. Prutting concluded her essay by stating:

> There are many levels of knowing. The promise in our sixth decade is for a renewed intellectual spirit in which it is realized that our understanding of an individual with a communicative disorder can only be as strong as our understanding of the basic tenets of science. (p. 262)

APPLICATIONS FROM THE HUMAN SCIENCES TO SUPERVISION

Perhaps because supervision is a relatively young specialization, it has not adhered rigidly to only one approach to knowing. Nevertheless, it has been influenced significantly by the logical positivist approach. This influence can be seen in concerns about accountability, objectivity, quantification, and cause–effect explanations. It can also be seen in the specification of tasks and competencies for both supervisors and students and in research based on a natural science paradigm.

Supervision has also been influenced by an interpretive-phenomenological approach to knowing, or what Prutting (1983) called the hermeneutic tradition in science. This influence can be seen in supervisors' interests in constructs based in counseling and interpersonal communication, in their concern about relationships and human growth, and in research based in the human sciences.

These two sets of influences have not been mutually exclusive in supervision. For example, a model of supervision that calls for quantification and measurement (Anderson, 1981) also stresses the need for human growth and values interpersonal interaction. A model of supervision that stresses empathic understanding (Caracciolo, Rigrodsky & Morrison, 1978) also stresses the need for operational definitions.

As Prutting (1983) asserted, both the hermeneutic and positivist traditions provide a base from which to work in Human Communication Disorders. Nevertheless, the human science tradition would appear to be the lesser known and understood of the two traditions. For this reason, and because both the human sciences and supervision are so clearly person-focused, this section explores three themes from an interpretive-phenomenological approach to knowing within the human sciences and relates them to supervision.

Interpretation

"Hermeneutics is the science of . . . interpretation" (Polkinghorne, 1983, p. 218) and probably originated in antiquity in the need to interpret sacred texts. For example, Biblical scholars continue to follow a set of interpretive rules (a hermeneutics) in studying both the Old and New Testaments. In the human science tradition, interpretive knowledge is what reveals human experience.

In daily communication, everyone applies interpretive rules in order to make sense of interactions. Interpretation has to do with the meanings that are created and assigned during interactions. Supervisors and student clinicians are constantly interpreting each other's as well as clients' emotions, physical states, motivations, and values. As health communication researchers, Kreps and Thornton (1984) stated, "Human beings have an insatiable appetite for creating meanings" (p. 21). On the other hand, there is a sense that interpretations need to be identified as such. Cole and Lacefield (1978), for example, in discussing skill domains for the helping professions, noted that "making observations, constructing inferences, and distinguishing between the two" is one of the critical skills helpers need to learn (p. 117). Similarly, the importance of identifying the frameworks — inferential sets — used for making interpretations and forming judgments has been stressed by writers such as Cogan (1973).

Interpretation is a key construct in the human sciences. When individuals interpret, they are engaging in a uniquely creative act, but an act that they never transcend fully; that is, individuals at some level are always part of what is being interpreted. The interpreter is not distinct from the interpreted or from the interpretation. This means that because the creative act is not transcendable, interpretation can never be "objective." As psychologist Mishler (1979) stated, "The perspective of the observer is intertwined with the phenomenon which does not have objective characteristics independent of the observer's perspective and methods" (p. 10). Truth, then, is relative to understanding (Lakoff & Johnson, 1980).

Human science acknowledges that statements are interpretable and data are constantly open to further interpretation and have no meaning if isolated from their interpreters. Human science acknowledges that interpretation, especially of interpersonal and communicative phenomena, is an ongoing human activity and an inescapable part of human experience.

Human science also acknowledges that guidelines for interpretation are needed (Polkinghorne, 1983). For example,

1. The phenomena interpreted should not be forced into preconceived interpretive schemes. Rather, the source of the interpreted meaning must be the phenomenon itself. In the supervisory process, this can mean trying to understand the significance of a particular therapeutic experience for a child, rather than interpreting the experience or behavior through the lens of, for example, the child's assumed need to control (a preconceived scheme).

2. The phenomena should not be interpreted solely in terms of their historical origins. In addition to those interpretations, the interpreter should determine the meaning for the present situation. In the supervisory process, this can mean attempting to understand the present meaning of a communicative disorder for a child, rather than focusing exclusively on its historical origins.

Attempting to understand the nature of interpretation, acknowledging the constancy of interpretation, and realizing that interpretations are not objective can lead supervisors to an enriched understanding of their interactions with students and students' interactions with clients. Interpretation, although not part of a model of science that values precision and lack of ambiguity, is part of a model of science — human science — that values understanding the character of the world as people experience it.

Accounts of Human Action

A question probed in depth in the human sciences, and the second theme to be explored here, concerns how to account for human action: Can it be accounted for by the same use of causal explanation present in the natural sciences? The human science tradition suggests that discussing human action, including human communication acts, from other than causal perspectives would enhance understanding of what human experience is about. Polkinghorne (1983) has discussed various theories that are available for understanding human action from other than traditional, deterministic notions of causality. Such theories acknowledge that "special qualities are involved in the understanding of human action" (Polkinghorne, 1983, p. 183). Thus, the human realm is acknowledged as having special characteristics. For example, because humans are reflective, there are dimensions to human action that do not correspond with any aspect of the rest of the biological and physical world.

Anthropologist Gregory Bateson (1972) probed causal questions of human action. He focused particularly on human communication and suggested that the world of communication and the world of physical occurrences are vastly different. It followed then that an approach to human communication action that was based on a view of linear causality (an identified antecedent-consequent relationship) was inappropriate. Pearce, Harris, and Cronen (1982) reported Bateson to be preoccupied with pattern and with interactions between persons. Such pattern perceiving is not congruent with simple causal accounts of human action. Hubbell (1981), in his application of Bateson's work to understanding causation within children's language disorders, argued that causation in human development is multiply determined and reciprocal (p. 120). He stressed the need to move away from "pat linear cause-and-effect explanations of causation" (p. 120).

One alternative to causal explanations is based in a teleological view of reality — teleology having to do with the purpose and function of a process or occurrence. This view suggests that exploring the purpose or function of human action is a more appropriate approach than looking for causal explanations. Teleological approaches to actions can lead to a focus on patterns over time and on the interactive system as a whole, as well as on its parts. Working with students to explore and understand the *function* a behavior or a pattern of behaviors has for them, the clients, or the relationship is different from probing for a causal explanation of the behavior. Hubbell (1981, chap. 5), in his work on children's language disorders, discussed the importance of a clinician attempting to determine the *function* of a client's behavior. He contrasted this approach with one that looks for a reason stemming from an internal state or emotion. For example, a child's expressions of anger could function to alter the therapist's interaction. Such an understanding by the clinician could be more helpful than speculating on the causes of the anger.

The human sciences suggest another alternative to causal explanation — one based in linguistic accounts in which the *nature* of statements is explored. This view asserts that when humans make statements that contain reasons for behavior, they are not offering explanations in the same way that explanations of natural events are offered.

According to Polkinghorne (1983, chap. 5), statements about reasons for action are really statements indicating that an individual is *accountable* for what has happened. For example, if a supervisor asks a student the reason why something was done, according to a linguistic-based view, the supervisor is really expecting the student to acknowledge intentionality and responsibility. In this view, both individuals in the interaction intuitively understand that *reasons* refer to aspects of their own interactions and not to a causal chain of events. An explanation, therefore, does not relate to information about acts, but to information about justification and responsibility (Polkinghorne, 1983, chap. 5).

Experience in clinical training suggests that both students and supervisors seek traditional causal explanations for clients' behaviors, including interpersonal behaviors. Applying ideas from the human sciences to human action would mean that supervisors and clinicians would begin to look at clinical (and supervisory) behaviors in ways that go beyond causal explanations. The behaviors could be looked at as part of a transactional system and as a way of functioning within that system. Such a view would go beyond the following kind of statement heard about a client: "Bobby just wasn't motivated."

Linguistic Expression

The third and last theme to be explored from the literature about interpretive-phenomenological approaches to knowing concerns human linguistic and communicative expression. "Access to the human realm is gained through its expressions" (Polkinghorne, 1983, p. 264). The human sciences make great use of linguistic expression during data collection, as exemplified by use of face-to-face interviews, written documents, discourse analysis, and oral narrative (storytelling).

If understanding the human realm is what the human sciences are about (and it is), if the human realm is one of meaning (and it is), and if humans communicate (and they do), studying communicative and linguistic expressions is probably the most appropriate way to understand human meaning. Such ideas are neither new nor surprising for supervisors who are constantly involved with human expression and linguistic data. On the other hand, supervisors may not have committed themselves to working with human expression and linguistic data in the supervisory process in ways that tap into the complexity and richness of those data. Learning that the human sciences and interpretive-phenomenological approaches truly value, study, and attempt to understand and find meaning in human expression can serve as a stimulus as well as a grounding for those persons who wish to probe supervisory and clinical linguistic data more fully than heretofore. Three aspects of human expression and linguistic data are commented on in this section.

Humans Use Metaphorical Language to Express Meaning

Hocker and Wilmot (1985), in their work on interpersonal conflict, noted that people often talk about conflict metaphorically. Examples they gave include "He shot down all my arguments" (the metaphor is that conflict is war) (p. 13), and "He's about to blow up" (the metaphor is that conflict is explosive) (p. 15). Other writers, such as Lakoff and Johnson (1980), have gone so far as to develop the thesis that the fundamental nature of humans' cognitive processes is metaphoric. They stated that "Metaphor is as much a part of our functioning as our sense of touch, and as precious" (p. 239).

According to Hocker and Wilmot (1985), metaphors function in at least three ways:

1. They give a synthesized, summarized view of a phenomenon.
2. They allow the expression of an experience that has no nomenclature.
3. They provide vivid imagery that evokes a strong experiential response.

Metaphors do not have to be a complete script; more often they simply provide cues to the speaker's meaning. Consider the following shared use of metaphor by a student and a supervisor when discussing a client's behavior:

> Student: I don't know. I really don't know what I think about it. I mean — I didn't like it. Um. It was — it was annoying. Sort of like — have you ever heard, like a faucet drip?
> Supervisor: And it won't stop, the damn thing!
> Student: Yea! Well, just that annoying — it just —
> Supervisor: Builds and builds until you reach a point — Damn faucet!
> Student: Yea! And so it's sort of like you grasp for, you know, whatever you think is going to work.
> Supervisor: Yup.

(Ellis, 1986)

Also consider the following metaphors used by a supervisor in talking to a student about a parent:

It gave her a plus and then zapped her, but it made the zap easier to take, I'm sure, for her. At least it would have if I were

Mrs. _____ I could swallow that. (Pickering, 1979, p. 374)

Both these excerpts were taken from transcripts that contained several more minutes of discourse. In neither transcript is there evidence that the metaphors were misunderstood by the communicative partner. The metaphors simply were part of the ongoing discourse. On the other hand, in neither transcript is there evidence that the affect represented in the metaphor was probed or that the metaphors were used as a source of analysis to understand dimensions of the interpersonal communication under discussion. For example, probing underlying meaning of the student's metaphor in the first example could lead into a discussion of how she views herself as a clinician — is it as someone who could *fix* the client's behavior if only she had the right tool?

Metaphors are part of the linguistic data of humans. Learning about their use and meaning in supervisory interactions could lead both supervisors and students to increased understanding of human linguistic expression.

Supervision is a Context for Metacommunication.

People talk to each other about their communication. Communication theorists such as Hocker and Wilmot (1985) define such communication about communication as metacommunication. Bateson (1972) described the metacommunicative level as the level used to "correct our perception of communicative behaviors" (p. 215). He stated that "In any normal relationship there is a constant interchange of metacommunicative messages such as 'What do you mean?' or 'Why did you do that?' ... and so on" (p. 215).

The supervisory process is one built on the assumptive value of metacommunication. As Naremore (1984) pointed out, the supervision conference is a place for participants to communicate about communication — the communication of the clinical process. In fact, Pickering (1984), in a study of conference interactions, found that "a major focus in the conferences was the clients and their progress" (p. 192). She reported further, however, that the discussions of interpersonal concerns involving clients did not include in-depth analyses of communicative dynamics. The findings of Roberts and Smith (1982) are also of interest here. In their study of supervisory conferences, they found that both supervisors and students used primarily simplistic rather than complex statements and primarily analytic rather than evaluative statements. These findings suggest that whatever the content of the interactions studied, the depth and professional sophistication with which the content was discussed were slight. Although no supervisory studies are known for which metacommunication per se is a variable, the two studies cited evoke a concern as to whether students and supervisors metacommunicate about the clinical process with a depth of analysis most beneficial for client change and student development.

Supervisors and students could also communicate about their communication with each other. They could talk about their roles, expectations, and needs in the relationship. In fact, Cogan (1973) and Goldhammer (1969) advocate such talk as part of Phase I of their Clinical Supervision Models. Moreover, supervisors and students could communicate about their own relational patterns with one another. Perhaps the participants do engage in such talk, but there are not enough data about supervisory discourse to know to what extent this is so. There is one report (Pickering, 1984) that indicates that supervisors consciously chose *not* to talk with students about aspects of their relationship. Communication scholars, on the other hand, suggest that metacommunication can lead to healthier relationships (Ruesch, 1973) and is a way of resolving relational conflict and breaking "the cycle of accusation, defense, and counteraccusation" (Wilmot, 1979, p. 194).

Communication scholars such as Rossiter (1974) also suggest that the ability to metacommunicate, that is, to describe and evaluate communication behaviors, can be developed. Metacommunication is a skill that both students and supervisors may need to learn. A caveat, however; talking about relational communication, if done without finesse, without positive intent, or without a concern for the partner's experience can lead to defensiveness, erosion of trust, and heightened anxiety about the self as well as about the process. The interpersonal communication literature thus contains suggestions that can enhance the ability to metacommunicate. For example, Smith and Williamson (1985) noted the importance of acknowledging another's communication, and Deetz and Stevenson (1986) discussed the helpfulness of using concrete descriptions. In addition, Wilmot (1979) identified the importance of *wanting* to break out of communicative cycles of misunderstanding and discord that damage relationships.

Supervision is a context for metacommunication, and the limitations on the richness of what is discussed come only from the participants themselves. The person-focused nature of the discourse, as well as of the process per se, suggest the importance of communicating about communication.

Language and Communication Have a Moral Dimension

Barnlund (1962), a communication scholar, noted that there is an inherent moral aspect in interpersonal communication. He discussed messages whose intent is to coerce or to exploit. Coercive communication means ignoring the values of the other person, and exploitive communication means subverting those values. Another choice, according to Barnlund, is to respect the values of the other, which means choosing facilitative communication. Certainly, all such choices are moral ones.

Laing (1967), noted for his work in disturbed and disturbing patterns of communication, has shown that through communication, individuals can be alienated from their own experience. He noted that in communicating with others, persons establish, lose, destroy, and regain relationships. This process suggests moral dimensions to the choices made when individuals communicate with each other.

In the supervisory process, choices are made about what to discuss, how to discuss it, and the supervisory model to follow. Choices are made as to what kind of communication to use to get the client (or student) to "comply." Choices are made as to whether to confirm the perceptions and inner experiences of the student (or client), to judge them negatively, to ignore them, or to turn them against the person. Furthermore, supervisors choose whether or not to show students sympathy, compassion, and understanding while these students are trying to fit themselves into the Procrustean bed of clinical intervention. Truly, communication in the supervisory setting has a moral dimension. Realizing this can be a first step toward leading both supervisors and students into communicative analyses that increasingly reflect the depth and complexity of human linguistic expression in both the clinical and supervisory process.

These three aspects of human linguistic expression — the presence of metaphor in communication, the place of metacommunication, and the moral dimension of communication — are but a sample of what exists to be explored in human communication. For example, the whole realm of nonverbal communication has not even been considered. Furthermore, the three themes from interpretive-phenomenological approaches to knowing discussed in this section — interpretation, approaches to human action, and linguistic expression — are only a sample of the themes discussed and explored in the human sciences.

The paradigm used to know the world, whether it be the physical or interpersonal worlds, or the clinical or supervisory worlds, will be an inescapable influence on what is seen, explored, interpreted, discussed, valued, and concluded.

SUMMARY AND CONCLUSIONS

To summarize this discussion, it is important to note that the literature provides ample evidence for contextualizing supervision as person-focused and that numerous parallels can be drawn between the clinical and supervisory processes. Considering the nature of the supervisory process leads to considering the paradigms used for knowing and understanding its multidimensional reality. In this chapter, two ways of knowing have been discussed — one based in the natural sciences, and one in the human sciences — and three themes from an interpretive-phenomenological approach to knowing have been presented. These themes — interpretation, accounts of human action, and linguistic expression — have been applied to supervision in Human Communication Disorders.

The implications arising from supervision being person-focused are numerous; five are discussed here.

One major implication is that the field would benefit from learning about the nature of supervisory relationships and supervisory interaction — not only *what* happens or should happen vis-à-vis a particular model, but also the *meaning* for the participants of what happens. It seems axiomatic that the participants would want to learn more about the meaning of this crucial professional relationship. A collateral implication is that the participants should be committed to increasing their knowledge about dyadic relational communication and about how to discuss and analyze dyadic relational communication — their own, but, perhaps more significantly, that which occurs in the clinical process. In such a regulated field, to have no required coursework on interpersonal communication theory or practice in ASHA certification requirements is to fail to acknowledge or validate the person-focused nature of the work.

A second major implication of supervision being person-focused is that supervision could benefit from having a dialectical relationship with the human sciences. Supervision could be enhanced by understanding what Prutting (1983) referred to as the hermeneutic tradition in scientific inquiry. The positivist approach has been a major influence and should not be lost. Nevertheless, there is much to learn about the nature of a human-oriented field by using approaches and constructs that both probe and originate in human experience. Supervision, as a field that involves both inquiry and practice, should learn its own experiential foundation, its own make-up. It must guard against being simply a derivative of something else, whether that something else is counseling or an aspect of the behavioral sciences. As a person-focused process, supervision can enhance its knowledge and understanding about what it is through probing and applying constructs from the human sciences.

A third major implication, or set of implications, is of a different sort and has to do with supervision being a person-focused specialty in an organizational setting — academe — where helping and helping professions are not usually part of the mainstream. For super visors, some of the outcomes of being outside the norm in academe include problems of salary, status, stratification, and workload (Gavett, 1985; Kennedy, 1985; Pickering, 1985; Rassi, 1985). There may also be interpersonal issues that arise out of encounters between individuals in a supervisory group that is largely master's degree level and female, and individuals in an academic group that is largely doctoral level and male. Combining variables of gender, academic degree, and professional or academic status suggests issues relating to power and marginality, among others. Thus, for the academic-based supervisor, being involved in a person-focused specialty area may mean coping with numerous issues only tangentially related to the supervisory process, but socially and experientially significant, nonetheless. Another issue in academe is that supervisors can become the institutionalized nurturers of the training programs. Such a role comes about because being person-focused can mean valuing and expressing supportive, nurturing, and collaborative behaviors. Related to this are academe's apparent values concerning competition and separation of rationality and affect. Important questions develop: How can sensitivity to a person-focused process and to collaboration be maintained in an environment that stresses objectification and competition? How can the work of supporting students — if this is a value — be shared by all those involved in their professional education?

Another implication is that being person-focused means taking an inter- or multidisciplinary approach to learning. Certainly the field of Human Communication Disorders has been exemplary in doing just that. On the other hand, there is a sense that the field is not offering its students as much involvement with the humanities as it might (Prutting, 1983). An interdisciplinary approach to learning suggests a pluralistic approach to knowing, that is, a realization that the world is too complex to understand on the basis of knowledge arising out of any one discipline or on the basis of an epistemology arising out of any one way of viewing the world. A person-focused process simply has too much ambiguity, change, complexity, and contradiction for the discipline, or the practitioner, to approach it from only one perspective. A caveat to this assertion is that the discipline and its practitioners must guard against a superficial, expedient, and ungrounded eclecticism.

A final implication of being person-focused is that because the human encounter is never value-free, supervision is not value-free. Values are employed continuously, from choices about models of inquiry for scholarly endeavors, to choices about ways of interpreting and understanding a client's behaviors during supervisory conference discussions. The question is not how to become value-*free*, but how to *identify and articulate those values* that inescapably guide choices. Even more importantly, because supervision is a teaching process, a vital consideration becomes: How can students be helped to examine their basic values regarding people, change, and human interaction?

Supervision as a person-focused process is both challenging and exciting. Perhaps one of the most exciting aspects is that supervision provides its participants with the opportunity to meet one another as thinking and feeling, growing and developing human beings. As Laing (1967) has stated, "We all live on the hope that authentic meeting between human beings can still occur" (pp. 26–27).

REFERENCES

Anderson, J. L. (1981). Training of supervisors in speech–language pathology and audiology. *Asha, 23*(2), 77–82.

Andreani, B. & Peters, M. (1977). *A supervisory process model in speech pathology.* Kent, OH: Department of Speech Pathology and Audiology.

Barnlund, D. C. (1962). Toward a meaning-centered philosophy of communication. *Journal of Communication, 12,* 197–211.

Bateson, G. (1972). *Steps to an ecology of mind.* New York: Ballantine Books.

Bender, H. E. (1975). Dilthey's voice in the emerging consciousness of humanistic education. *Journal of Education* (Boston University), *157*(2), 31–43.

Berger, P. L. & Luckmann, T. (1966). *The social construction of reality.* Garden City, NY: Doubleday.

Berman, M. (1981). *The reenchantment of the world.* Ithaca, NY: Cornell University Press.

Brammer, L. M. (1985). *The helping relationship* (3rd ed.). Englewood Cliffs, NJ: Prentice-Hall.

Brasseur, J. A. & Anderson, J. L. (1983). Observed differences between direct, indirect, and direct/indirect videotaped supervisory conferences. *Journal of Speech and Hearing Research, 26,* 349–355.

Capra, F. (1982). *The turning point.* New York: Simon & Schuster.

Caracciolo, G. L., Rigrodsky, S. & Morrison, E. B. (1978). A Rogerian orientation to the speech–language pathology supervisory relationship. *Asha, 20,* 286–290.

Chubrich, R. E. (1978). Session obsession: A former client looks at therapy. *Journal of National Student Speech and Hearing Association, 6,* 70–78.

Cogan, M. L. (1973). *Clinical supervision.* Boston, MA: Houghton Mifflin.

Cole, H. P. & Lacefield, W. E. (1978). Skill domains critical to the helping professions. *Personnel and Guidance Journal, 57*(2), 115–123.

Coles, R. (1979). Medical ethics and living a lie. *The New England Journal of Medicine, 301*(8), 444–446.

Cooper, E. R., Boone, D. R., Murphy, A. T., Knepflar, K. J., Rees, N. S. & VanHattum, R. J. (1982, November). *The client–clinician relationship in speech and language therapy: The undefined variable.* Paper presented at the meeting of the American Speech–Language–Hearing Association, Toronto, Ontario, Canada.

Darroch, V. & Silvers, R. J. (Eds.). (1982). *Interpretive human studies: An introduction to phenomenological research.* Washington, DC: University Press of America.

Deetz, S. A. & Stevenson, S. L. (1986). *Managing interpersonal communication.* New York: Harper & Row, Publishers.

Donovan, J. (1985). *Feminist theory: The intellectual traditions of American feminism.* New York: Frederick Ungar.

Dowling, S. & Wittkopp, J. (1982). Students' perceived supervisory needs. *Journal of Communication Disorders, 15,* 319–328.

Eisenstein, H. (1983). *Contemporary feminist thought.* Boston, MA: G. K. Hall.

Eisenstein, Z. R. (1981). *The radical future of liberal feminism.* Boston, MA: Northeastern University Press.

Ellis, L. (1986, November). *An approach to supervisor self-confrontation.* Paper presented at the meeting of the American Speech–Language–Hearing Association, Detroit, MI.

Emerick, L. L. & Hood, S. B. (Eds.). (1974). *The client–clinician relationship.* Springfield, IL: Charles C Thomas.

Fey, M. E. (1986). *Language intervention with young children.* San Diego, CA: College-Hill Press.

Gavett, E. (1985). Competencies, qualifications, training: Speech–language pathology. In J. E. Bernthal (Ed.), *Proceedings of the Sixth Annual Conference on Graduate Education* (pp. 20–25). Lincoln, NE: University of Nebraska, Council of Graduate Programs in Communication Sciences and Disorders.

Gildston, P. & Gildston, H. (1972). An existential approach to speech therapy. *Journal of Communication Disorders, 5,* 32–38.

Goldhammer, R. (1969). *Clinical supervision.* New York: Holt-Rinehart-Winston.

Ham, R. (1986). *Techniques of stuttering therapy.* Englewood Cliffs, NJ: Prentice-Hall.

Hess, C. W. (1976). Language intervention with children: A goal-oriented approach. *Journal of the National Student Speech and Hearing Association, 4,* 32–39.

Hocker, J. L. & Wilmot, W. W. (1985). *Interpersonal conflict* (2nd ed.). Dubuque, IA: Wm. C. Brown.

Hubbell, R. D. (1981). *Children's language disorders.* Englewood Cliffs, NJ: Prentice-Hall.

Johnson, A. R., Prudhomme, M. R. & Rogero, E. A. (1982). Competency-based objectives for the student teaching experience. *Language, Speech, and Hearing Services in Schools, 13,* 187–196.

Kamhi, A. G. (1984). Problem-solving in child language disorders: The clinician as clinical scientist. *Language, Speech, and Hearing Services in Schools, 15,* 226–234.

Kennedy, K. (1985). Hidden dynamics related to the supervisory role. In J. E. Bernthal (Ed.), *Proceedings of the Sixth Annual Conference of Graduate Education* (pp. 33–39). Lincoln, NE: University of Nebraska, Council of Graduate Programs in Communication Sciences and Disorders.

Kreps, G. L. & Thornton, B. C. (1984). *Health communication.* New York: Longman.

Laing, R. D. (1967). *The politics of experience.* New York, Patheon Books, A Division of Random House.

Lakoff, G. & Johnson, M. (1980). *Metaphors we live by.* Chicago, IL: The University of Chicago Press.

Lerner, G. (1979). *The majority finds its past: Placing women in history.* New York: Oxford University Press.

McCrea, E. S. (1980). Supervisee ability to self-explore and four facilitative dimensions of supervisor behavior in individual conferences in speech-language pathology (Doctoral dissertation, Indiana University, 1980). *Dissertation Abstracts International, 41*(06), 2134-B. (University Microfilms No. 80-29, 239).

McKerrow, R. E. (1980, November). *Validating arguments: A phenomenological perspective.* Paper presented at the meeting of the Speech Communication Association, New York.

Martin, E. W. (1963). Client-centered therapy as a theoretical orientation for speech therapy. *Asha, 5,* 576–578.

Maslow, A. H. (1966). *The psychology of science: A reconnaissance.* Chicago, IL: Henry Regnery Company.

Mishler, E. G. (1979). Meaning in context: Is there any other kind? *Harvard Educational Review, 49*(1), 1–19.

Morgan, R. (1984). *The anatomy of freedom: Feminism, physics and global politics.* Garden City, NY: Anchor Books/Doubleday.

Murphy, A. T. (1974). The quiet hyena: Two monologues in search of a dialogue. In L. L. Emerick & S. B. Hood (Eds.), *The client–clinician relationship* (pp. 29–44). Springfield, IL: Charles C Thomas.

Murphy, A. (1982). The clinical process and the speech–language pathologist. In G. H. Shames & E. H. Wiig (Eds.), *Human communication disorders: An introduction* (pp. 453–474). Columbus, OH: Charles E. Merrill.

Murphy, A. T. (1985, March). Research in special education: Traditional and non-traditional. In *Update of Research in Special Education.* Symposium conducted at Boston University, Boston, MA.

Naremore, R. C. (1984, November). Discussion. In J. L. Anderson (Chair), *Research methodologies for the supervisory process.* Double miniseminar presented at the meeting of the American Speech–Language–Hearing Association, San Francisco, CA.

Oratio, A. R. (1977). *Supervision in speech pathology: A handbook for supervisors and clinicians.* Baltimore, MD: University Park Press.

Pearce, W. B., Harris, L. M. & Cronen, V. E. (1982). Communication theory in a new key. In C. Wilder and J. H. Weakland (Eds.), *Rigor and imagination: Essays from the legacy of Gregory Bateson* (pp. 149–194). New York: Praeger.

Perkins, W. H. (1971). *Speech pathology: An applied behavioral science.* St. Louis, MO: C. V. Mosby.

Pickering, M. (1977). An examination of concepts operative in the supervisory process and relationship. *Asha, 19,* 607–610.

Pickering, M. (1979). Interpersonal communication in speech–language pathology clinical practicum: A descriptive, humanistic perspective (Doctoral dissertation, Boston University, 1979). *Dissertation Abstracts International, 40,* 2140-41B. (University Microfilms No. 79-23, 892).

Pickering, M. (1981, November). *Supervisory interaction: The subjective side.* Paper presented for the program of the Council of University Supervisors of Practicum in Speech–Language Pathology and Audiology, Los Angeles, CA.

Pickering M. (1984). Interpersonal communication in speech–language pathology supervisory conferences: A qualitative study. *Journal of Speech and Hearing Disorders, 49,* 189–195.

Pickering, M. (1985). Clinical supervision in a university setting: Overview of the Topic. In J. E. Bernthal (Ed.), *Proceedings of the Sixth Annual Conference on Graduate Education* (pp. 15–19). Lincoln, NE: University of Nebraska, Council of Graduate Programs in Communication Sciences and Disorders.

Pickering, M. & McCready, V. (1983). Supervisory journals: An 'inside' look at supervision. *SUPERvision, 7*(1), 5–7 (Summary).

Polkinghorne, D. (1983). *Methodology for the human sciences: Systems of inquiry.* Albany, NY: State University of New York Press.

Prutting, C. A. (1983). Scientific inquiry and communicative disorders: An emerging paradigm across six decades. In T. M. Gallagher & C. A. Prutting (Eds.), *Pragmatic assessment and intervention issues in language* (pp. 247–266). San Diego, CA: College-Hill Press.

Rassi, J. (1985). Competencies, qualifications, training: Audiology. In J. E. Bernthal (Ed.), *Proceedings of the Sixth Annual Conference on Graduate Education* (pp. 26–32). Lincoln, NE: University of Nebraska, Council of Graduate Programs in Communication Sciences and Disorders.

Rich, A. (1976). *Of woman born: Motherhood as experience and institution.* New York: W. W. Norton.

Roberts, J. E. & Smith, K. J. (1982). Supervisor–supervisee role differences and consistency of behavior in supervisory conferences. *Journal of Speech and Hearing Research, 25,* 428–434.

Rossiter, C. M., Jr. (1974). Instruction in metacommunication. *Central States Speech Journal, 25,* 36–42.

Ruesch, J. (1973). *Therapeutic communication* (2nd ed.). New York: W. W. Norton.

Ruether, R. R. (1975). *New woman/new earth: Sexist ideologies and human liberation.* New York: The Seabury Press, Inc.

Schoenberg, M.C., Larson, L. C. & Gevaart, C. C. (1980–1981). The Schoenberg parametric model of supervision. *SUPERvision, 4*(4), 23–27 (Summary).

Shearer, W. M. (1982). *Research procedures in speech, language, and hearing.* Baltimore, MD: Williams & Wilkins.

Shriberg, L.D., Filley, F. S., Hayes, D. M., Kwiatkowski, J., Schatz, J. A., Simmons, K. M. & Smith, M. E. (1975). The Wisconsin procedure for appraisal of clinical competence (W-PACC): Model and data. *Asha, 17,* 158–165.

Siegel, G. M. & Spradlin, J. E. (1985). Therapy and research. *Journal of Speech and Hearing Disorders, 50,* 226–230.

Silverman, F. H. (1985). *Research design and evaluation in speech pathology and audiology* (2nd ed.). Englewood Cliffs, NJ: Prentice-Hall.

Smith, D. R. & Williamson, L. K. (1985). *Interpersonal communication: Roles, rules, strategies, and games* (3rd ed.). Dubuque, IA: Wm. C. Brown.

Smith, K. J. & Anderson, J. L. (1982). Relationship of perceived effectiveness to verbal interaction/content variables in supervisory conferences in speech–language pathology. *Journal of Speech and Hearing Research, 25,* 252–261.

Spender, D. (1980). *Man made language.* Boston, MA: Routledge & Kegan Paul.

Thomas, E. J. (1984). *Designing interventions for the helping professions.* Beverly Hills, CA: Sage Publications, Inc.

Thorne, B., Kramarae, C. & Henley, N. (1983). *Language, gender, and society.* Rowley, MA: Newbury House.

Travis, L. E. (Ed.). (1957). *Handbook of speech pathology.* New York: Appleton–Century–Crofts.

Van Riper, C. (1965). Supervision of clinical practice. *Asha, 7,* 75–77.

Volz, H. B., Klevans, D. R., Norton, S. J. & Putens, D. L. (1978). Interpersonal communication skills of speech–language pathology undergraduates: The effects of training. *Journal of Speech and Hearing Disorders, 43,* 524–542.

Ward, L. M. & Webster, E. J. (1965). The training of clinical personnel: I. Issues in conceptualization. *Asha, 7,* 38–40.

Wilmot, W. W. (1979). *Dyadic communication* (2nd ed.). Reading, MA: Addison-Wesley.

Wolf, F. A. (1981). *Taking the quantum leap.* New York: Harper & Row.

Wollman, I. L. & Conover, H. B. (1979). The student clinician's perception of the supervisory process. *Ohio Journal of Speech and Hearing, 14,* 192–201.

PART III:

Interpersonal Perspectives

CHAPTER 6

Supervision and Self-Exploration

Martha B. Crago

T he crucial role of self-examination in supervision is indicated by the American Speech–Language–Hearing Association's position paper on Clinical Supervision in Speech–Language Pathology and Audiology (ASHA, 1985):

> A central premise of supervision is that effective clinical teaching involves in a fundamental way the development of self-analysis, self-evaluation, and problem-solving on the part of the individual being supervised. The success of clinical teaching rests largely on the achievement of this goal. (p. 57)

Self-examination, that is, self-analysis and self-evaluation, takes many forms. This chapter focuses on self-exploration. In the first half of the chapter, the concept of self-exploration is introduced, pertinent literature is reviewed, and the importance of self-exploration to the supervisor is discussed. In the second half of the chapter, a self-exploratory training model for supervision is described.

SELF-EXPLORATION IN SUPERVISION

Self-examination as it relates to supervision in Human Communication Disorders and other fields has been referred to by a number of terms, among them self-awareness (Kaplan & Dreyer, 1974), self-evaluation (Anderson, 1981), self-critiquing (Bernstein & Lecomte,

1976), and self-analysis (Anderson, 1981). The term *self-exploration* is used in this chapter because it has two meanings. One meaning has to do with looking inward at an individual's behaviors, at process dynamics, and at interactions. The other meaning has to do with changing behavior and moving ahead. The explorations associated with the second meaning are based on the explorations associated with the first meaning. Self-exploration implies both an inward, detailed, search-and-find process of analysis and an outward, pushing forward process of discovery into new uncharted ways of behaving. Self-exploration is a skill that is developed in students during supervision. Its use does not end at the completion of a university degree, but rather extends into professional life. The ability to analyze one's functioning and determine a route for desired change is an essential skill for becoming and remaining a competent professional. It is, likewise, fundamentally important for the growth and development of the supervisor.

Self-exploration in supervision means using the self in a meaningful and knowledgeable way. Using the self as a source of information and change leads to an internalization of supervision. Throughout their careers, supervisees (either students or professionals) can use self-exploration as a means for acquiring knowledge and for effecting change in themselves.

It is the premise of this chapter that self-exploration is an important and central skill in Human Communication Disorders supervision.

Relevant Supervisory Models and Pertinent Research

A variety of fields in addition to Human Communication Disorders, including Social Work, Counseling Psychology, and Psychiatry, have discussed self-exploration in their literature. In this section of the chapter, we will highlight this literature and underline its relevance to a supervisory training program in speech–language pathology.

The literature from Human Communication Disorders will be examined first. There are two models of supervision (Anderson, 1980; Oratio, 1977) and one research study (McCrea, 1980) in which the authors have dealt with concepts associated with what is referred to in this chapter as self-exploration. Of these three authors, only McCrea used the specific term self-exploration. The McGill University training program described later in this chapter puts into practice several aspects of Oratio's and Anderson's models and draws on the implications of McCrea's research.

Oratio (1977) proposed a transactive model of supervision that integrated cognitive, emotional, and experiential elements of the supervisory process and stressed the importance of what he referred to as self-supervision. In Oratio's model, the student becomes self-supervising by a gradual process that includes observation by the supervisor, post-therapy conferencing, analysis of therapy, and simulated single skill practice. These activities are structured to facilitate the eventual aim of becoming self-supervising.

Anderson applied the Clinical Supervision Model derived from Cogan (1973) and Goldhammer (1969) to Human Communication Disorders. In the Clinical Supervision Model, the development of a self-supervising student is a primary concern of the supervisor. The supervisor and supervisee, jointly, are responsible for planning, observation, and analysis of the observation, as well as joint collaboration on the supervisory conference. Anderson (1980) stated:

> This partnership, according to the proponents of Clinical Supervision, leads to a more analytical, problem-solving and, ultimately, self-supervising supervisee. The methodology excludes the possibility of the supervisor as a superior member in a superior–subordinate relationship where the supervisor's role is perceived to be that of the authority figure who determines, directs and evaluates the supervisee's behavior based on his/her own biases and perceptions only. (p. 1)

Like Oratio, Anderson described the end product of supervision as a self-supervising clinician. Self-reliance becomes an outcome of self-supervision. It provides the clinician with an essential skill for developing and maintaining professional competency. Its importance to the clinician led Anderson (1981) to list teaching "supervisees the technique of self-analysis and self-evaluation" (p. 81) as one of her eight clinical teaching (supervision) competencies.

McCrea (1980) studied the effects of four supervisory behaviors: *empathic understanding, respect, facilitative genuineness,* and *concreteness of expression* on the supervisee's self-exploratory behavior. Empathic understanding and respect were significant predictors of supervisee self-exploration. An increase in these behaviors could then be presumed to lead to an increase in self-exploration. Indeed, such an increase would seem warranted, since only nine percent of the supervisee's utterances in McCrea's study were found to be self-exploratory. Only one percent of the supervisor's utterances were coded as empathic understanding. McCrea's work suggests the need for the kind of training program in speech–language pathology supervision that is addressed in this chapter.

Interest in concepts related to self-exploration is apparent in the literature of other professional fields. In the field of Counseling Psychology, there are descriptions of training programs in supervision, developmental models of supervision, and supervisory research that have relevance to self-exploration.

Kagan (1975) developed a systematic procedure by which students in Counseling Psychology could learn to self-explore. His Interpersonal Process Recall Model stresses self-evaluation based on focused self-observation. He made systematic use of videotapes so that students and clients might understand themselves better, recognize their impact on others, and realize the impact of others on them. He found that by using respectful inquiry after a counseling session, there was an increase in participant awareness and taking responsibility for feelings. In addition, the trainees were better able to self-analyze and self-critique. Their insights about and motivation to change also improved.

Similarly, Bernstein and Lecomte (1976, 1979) recognized the need for a training procedure whose stated goal was the development of student self-reliance. Bernstein and Lecomte's basic assumption was that skills in self-evaluation are crucial to the development of a competent professional. Furthermore, they asserted that these skills could be learned. To this end, Bernstein and Lecomte developed a training protocol that integrated the cognitive and experiential elements of learning in a systematic step-by-step procedure.

The supervisory training in speech–language pathology described later in this chapter is similar in many respects to Bernstein and Lecomte's protocol. For this reason, it is instructive to review their experiences in developing what they referred to as the ability to self-critique. Bernstein and Lecomte's counseling students made presentations of self-selected, self-evaluated videotaped excerpts for comparison with trained supervisor's assessments of the same segments. The level of congruence between the two determined the students' ability to self-evaluate. Bernstein and Lecomte found that prior to systematic self-critique training, their students' self-evaluations were ill-focused and represented global emotionally based responses. With increased use of the technique, trainees were able to articulate their evaluations more clearly. Beginning level counselors found it difficult to discriminate between more and less effective responses and to provide reasons for their responses. Their ability to present a cogent rationale for their responses increased with time. Furthermore, the authors stated that the development of a personal counseling style was facilitated by the opportunity to view, in a supervision group, a variety of effective and less effective approaches to similar clients.

Littrell, Lee-Borden, and Lorenz (1979), also writing in the area of counselor training, presented ideas that are important to consider in Human Communication Disorders supervision training. They incorporated four separate but related models of counselor supervision into a unified process with a developmental framework. The emphasis is on the developmental stages through which a trainee passes. In their framework, each stage is associated with a model of supervision. It is at the final stage that the supervisee is ready for the self-supervising model.

> The distinguishing feature of Stage IV, the self-supervising model, is that the counselor becomes the principal designer of his or her learning. Upon reaching this stage, the conceptualization, implementation, control, and management of supervision are the counselor's responsibilities as a professional. (p. 134)

Littrell and colleagues (1979) pointed out that models and programs to implement self-supervision were receiving increased attention. They stressed that studies of these programs needed to be made in order to establish their effectiveness and suggested that the following specific features be researched: induction of change, generalization across situations, and maintenance over time.

The research of Robinson, Kurpius, and Froehle (1979) substantiated the viability and desirability of encouraging students to generate self-exploration and self-analysis of their performance. These authors demonstrated that counselor trainees could evaluate their own behavior. Self-generated performance feedback by the trainees was compared to expert performance feedback and to no performance feedback. Results of this study showed that those trainees who received feedback outperformed the controls who received no feedback. Nevertheless, there was no significant difference between the two sources of performance feedback. Furthermore, those trainees who generated their own feedback reported high levels of satisfaction with this approach to learning basic skills.

Writing in the field of Social Work, Lowy (1983) identified models of supervision used in his field. His work, too, has application to Human Communications Disorders supervision. He addressed the learning and teaching process of supervision. Self-reliance, according to Lowy, should be developed in the social work trainee by encouraging self-exploration. He described supervision as involving adult learners who have accumulated certain life experiences. Adult learners, he said, could utilize their experiences to a maximum if they were allowed to evaluate their already formed ideas and responses in an atmosphere of mutual sharing and nonthreatening give and take. Lowy found that adult learners responded most favorably to situations in which they could actively participate. Involvement in planning, designing, and implementing programs was suggested.

Adults were resistant to learning in situations that they viewed as incongruent to their self-autonomy.

In summary, there is a substantial amount of interest in the concept of self-exploration that has been expressed in a variety of fields. Models have placed self-exploration in an important position in the supervisory process. Research has substantiated the desirability of self-exploration for students but has found it to be infrequent in occurrence. Training procedures designed to increase self-exploratory skills have been posited. The effectiveness of these training procedures remains to be researched.

Self-Exploration and Growth for the Supervisor

Supervision is a mutual process involving both students and supervisors. The training model described later in this chapter considers both of these groups of people. The process of change should not be restricted to the students or trainees. In an interactional exchange, both supervisors and students can be expected to grow and develop in their professional skills. Supervisors can benefit from self-evaluation. To accomplish this, supervisors need to develop the same basic skills of self-exploration as their supervisees.

Lack of self-awareness in the supervisor can have serious consequences on the supervisory process. Stresses and strains exist in the supervisory process. Unresolved dilemmas can impede communication and growth for both students and supervisors. Yet, there is little institutionalized framework and support for developing and maintaining supervisory self-awareness. Gizynski (1978), writing in the field of Social Work, pointed out that supervisors need skills and training in self-awareness. She cited examples of the supervisor who had difficulty in responding appropriately to the student's dependency demands in supervision, the supervisor who was threatened by students whose character styles were different from her own, and the supervisor who viewed client behavior from a value system different from her student's value system. Other "hidden" dynamics are discussed by McCready, Shapiro, and Kennedy in Chapter 7 of this book. To perform adequately as a supervisor, a level of self-awareness is expected. A key to the discovery of problematic dynamics may be the development of adequate skills in self-exploration.

As a two-party transaction, supervision can be seen as a form of resource collaboration. This term is used by Tyler, Pargament, and Gatz (1983) to describe an interactional model of psychology that views expert-nonexpert interactions as involving a reciprocity of influence. In their model, "all participants acknowledge their own and each other's resources and recognize their reciprocal gain" (p. 388). This same concept is summed up in Lowy's (1983) phrase "teachers learn and learners teach" (p. 58). The concept that both supervisees and supervisors have something to offer each other implies that both parties have resources and deficits. Both the helper (supervisor) and helpee (supervisee) are capable of evaluating the relationship. Both gain from the interaction, and both change.

The supervision model that Anderson (1980) in Human Communication Disorders has adapted from Cogan (1973) and Goldhammer (1969) has colleagueship as a major guiding principle and goal. Supervisees and supervisors participate in a partnership. This model assumes that supervisors will analyze their behaviors in much the same way that supervisees do. Through analysis and the process of self-exploration, supervisors can grow professionally.

STUDENT–SUPERVISOR INTERACTIONAL SELF-EXPLORATORY TRAINING: THE MCGILL UNIVERSITY APPROACH

A protocol for self-exploration training within the context of speech–language pathology supervision was developed at McGill University. That protocol, Student–Supervisor Interactional Self-Exploratory Training, is described in this section. As the title implies, the training is for both students and supervisors. It is designed to improve and capitalize on the interaction of these two parties and to develop their abilities to self-explore.

Background

McGill University's School of Human Communication Disorders is small and is exclusively at the graduate level of training. Approximately eight students in speech–language pathology are graduated each year. The students have five supervisory experiences over their two years in the master's program. Because there is no university clinic, all practica and the final three-month internship take place in external clinical sites. The supervisors in these settings receive no monetary compensation for the time they spend supervising. They voluntarily attend courses and workshops on supervision at McGill free of charge. These courses and workshops have been offered at McGill University since 1980. The workshops on supervision took place in three different years (1980, 1981, and 1985). The course for supervisors, Supervision for Supervisors, was offered in 1982. It met once a month in the evenings over the academic year. In 1983 and 1984, the joint student–supervisor training sessions met regularly during the academic year.

Master's degree students take Practicum Preparation I, followed the next year by Practicum Preparation II. Each of these three-credit courses is taught by the practicum coordinator in speech–language pathology. The two courses differ in content. In the first year, students are introduced to basic clinical skills in speech–language pathology by discussing a series of videotapes (Crago, 1982) that have applicability to their off-campus practica. In Practicum Preparation II, students make tapes of their own clinical encounters and present them in class or in joint supervisor–student groups.

All speech–language pathology students also take a required six-credit course entitled Counseling and Supervision. This course spans both the first and second years. It is taught by a counseling psychologist who has specialized in supervision. In the first year, the Counseling and Supervision course introduces the students to interpersonal skills and attitudes as well as to some basic strategies associated with supervision. In the second year, interpersonal skills and attitudes are practiced by role-playing in class and by making tapes of counseling sessions with clients for presentation in class.

Training Protocols

Academic teaching at the university level characteristically uses a didactic approach. Conversely, clinical training is an experiential phenomenon. For this reason, Student Supervisor Interactional Self-Exploratory Training uses an experiential method of training clinical and supervisory skills. Concepts being taught are tried out in the classroom and in the clinic.

There are four major content areas in Student–Supervisor Self-Exploratory Training: goal specification, tape analysis, interpersonal skills, and feedback. Training in these four areas is described in the following sections.

Training in Goal Specification

At McGill University, the concept of goal specification is presented to the students in their Counseling and Supervision course. Actual practice in this skill takes place in Practicum Preparation courses.

Goal specification has been addressed in supervision literature from related disciplines. Littrell and colleagues (1979) described goal-setting as the first stage of the supervisory process. It represented the initial contact between supervisor and student and was the beginning of their joint venture. In psychiatry supervision, Goldberg (1985) discussed the need to respect individual variation. He cautioned that it is unlikely (and undesirable) for supervisors to move to uniform prescriptions about what, when, and how to teach. Yet, he suggested that general guiding principles for supervision, such as goal specification or, as Fox (1983) referred to it, contracting, can be beneficial. Fox defined the contract as an overt agreement between a student and a supervisor.

The specification of goals by a supervisee is the initial step in self-reliance. The supervisor draws the student's attention to relevant competencies and, by necessity, must represent her agency's, her clients', and her own personal needs. The students describe antecedent experiences and define the areas in which they are seeking to develop both personally and professionally. Students and supervisors can act as resources for each other in the process of goal specification. They stimulate one another's interest and clinical concerns. Supervisors also contract with supervisees for feedback on and discussion of their supervisory capabilities. Supervision based on specific goals, thus, has a clearly articulated sense of direction and purpose.

In Student-Supervisor Interactional Self-Exploratory Training, both students and supervisors are taught to specify goals by writing a contract. Students are shown a videotape entitled *Contracting* (Crago, 1982). This tape shows supervisee–supervisor pairs in the process of specifying practicum goals. In Practicum Preparation class, students role-play the situation of drawing up a contract before they make a contract with each of their supervisors. Supervisors in their course and workshops also learn how to develop a contract with a student. This is done by role-play situations and watching the *Contracting* videotape. An example of a contract written by a first-year master's student and her supervisor appears in Appendix A.

Training in Tape Analysis

Self-image confrontation using videotapes has been described in the literature from fields other than Human Communication Disorders. Kagan (1975), for instance, reported its use in counseling supervision. More recently, Froehle (1984), in that same field, integrated videotapes and computers for rapid data counting and analysis. In social work supervision, Star (1977) studied the effectiveness of videotape self-image confrontation on helping perceptions. Her results indicated that self-image confrontation produced significant amounts of perceptual change. Although the initial impact was powerful, the effects of single self-image confrontation tended to decrease over time. Star's findings suggested that effective use of videotapes required periodic and varied self-encounters throughout clinical training. Goldberg (1985) delineated the unique kinds of information that resulted from audio- versus videotaping in psychotherapy supervision.

Tape analysis is central to Student-Supervisor Interactional Self-Exploratory Training. A specific procedure for analyzing a video- or audiotape is used. Supervisees follow the guidelines found in Appendix B in preparing for supervision. These guidelines center on the following:

1. Self-selection of a tape segment
2. Self-analysis of the segment
3. Presentation of the segment to a supervisor
4. Resolving incongruent evaluations
5. Formulating alternatives
6. Analyzing the supervisory session
7. Formulating alternatives for future supervisory sessions

A set of guidelines for supervisors is found in Appendix C. At McGill University, there are three situations for tape analysis: student training, supervisory training, and joint group training. Each of these situations is described below.

STUDENT TRAINING. Students at McGill University learn to analyze tapes in the second year of the Practicum Preparation course. The protocol for this part of the course is outlined in Figure 6–1.
Students begin by taping a clinical encounter. The tape is then analyzed using at least two of the following analysis systems: Boone and Prescott (1972), Clezy Adaptation (Crago, 1980), Speech Act Analysis System (Becker & Silverstein, 1983), as well as the McGill Guidelines for Tape Analysis (Crago, 1983).

When students present their tapes in class, they are supervised by their peer group following an adapted format of Dowling's Teaching Clinic (1979). A group monitor is assigned to transcribe or tape the peer group supervision. This monitor then analyzes the supervisory process using one of the following supervisory analysis systems: Culatta and Seltzer (1976, 1977), Oratio (1979), or McCrea (1980). When the group monitor's analysis is completed, the peer group

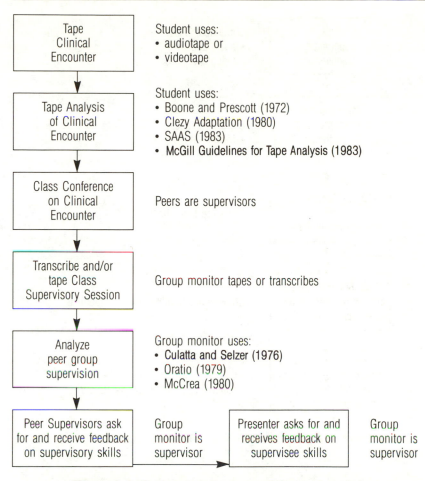

Figure 6–1. Student training protocol for tape analysis.

supervisors ask her for feedback on their supervisory skills. The student who presented the original tape asks for feedback on her supervisee skills. In this way, students learn both to self-explore and facilitate self-exploration.

In their practica, students prepare tapes of their clinical work. They present these tapes to their clinical supervisors following the guidelines previously explained for tape analysis. It is expected that students will analyze and present tapes on a regular basis in each of their clinical training sites.

SUPERVISOR TRAINING. The protocol for the supervisors' training in tape analysis is shown in Figure 6–2. For their course on supervision,

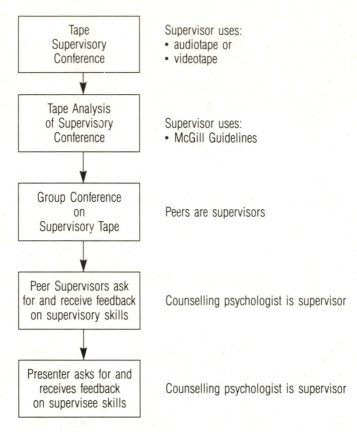

Figure 6–2. *Supervisor training protocol for tape analysis.*

supervisors made tapes of their supervisory conferences for presentation. The supervisors' tapes were analyzed and presented to a group of fellow professionals following the McGill Guidelines. While presenting and analyzing their tapes, the supervisors were in the role of supervisee. Their analysis and self-exploration were focused on the supervisory encounter. Peer group members were in the role of supervisors to the presenter and practiced their skills of facilitating self-exploration. The peer supervisors solicited and received feedback on *their* supervisory skills from the instructor of the supervisor's course.

JOINT TRAINING. Tapes were also made by student–supervisor pairs. These tapes were jointly analyzed and presented for feedback to a group of students and supervisors. This protocol is depicted in

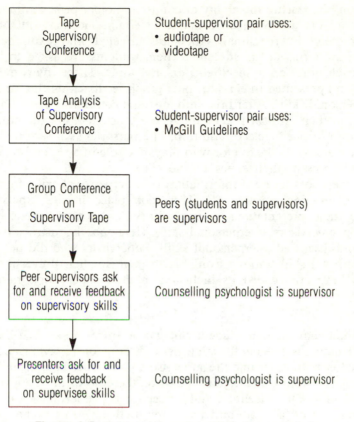

Figure 6–3. Joint training protocol for tape analysis.

Figure 6–3. The presenters were in the role of supervisees. The peer group members were in the role of supervisors. Both the skills of self-exploration and facilitation of self-exploration were practiced by students and supervisors.

Training in Interpersonal Skills

Interpersonal skill training for students takes place in their Counseling and Supervision course. The facilitator is a counseling psychologist whose training was based in Rogers (1961) and Carkhuff (1969a, 1969b). The course stresses active listening and the use of communicative behaviors associated with good listening (paraphrasing, reflecting feelings, and clarifying). This counseling psychologist also discusses concepts of empathy, genuineness, and respect. In addition, she teaches the ability to confront another person without affront and the ability to be concrete in communicating with others.

Initially, interpersonal skills are targeted and explained in behavioral terms to the students. Then, students are asked to interview each other on a specified personal topic. These interviews are taped and presented in class for peer group feedback on the student's interpersonal skills. After this, students tape counseling sessions with clients in their clinical practicum. These tapes, too, are presented to the group for feedback. In addition, interpersonal skills are modeled for the class by the instructor who plays the role of a supervisor when students present their tapes to the class.

Supervisors received information on interpersonal skills from the same counseling psychologist. This took place in the supervisors' course. Tape presentations of supervisory conferences were used to develop supervisors' interpersonal skills. Here, too, the instructor modeled and discussed interpersonal skills. Supervisors who did not have interpersonal skill training available to them in their university programs have appreciated its inclusion in their supervisory training.

Training in Feedback

Additional time in Student Supervisor Interactional Self-Exploratory Training is given to the strategies of asking for, receiving, and giving feedback. In order that the supervisory conference be a meaningful exchange between student and supervisor, there needs to be a give and take of information, feelings, and perceptions. The feedback strategies are designed to facilitate and make more effective this exchange between student and supervisor. There are guidelines for asking, giving, and receiving feedback in Appendices C, D, and E of this chapter. These guidelines are designed for both supervisees and supervisors. Supervisees ask for and receive feedback, as well as give feedback to each of their supervisors. Although supervisors often give feedback, they also ask for and receive it from both students and peers.

A videotape on *Feedback* (Crago, 1982) is shown to students in their Counseling and Supervision course. Supervisors were introduced to feedback strategies in their course. Role-play exercises on giving, receiving, and asking for feedback were a part of that course. Feedback skills are further developed by the in-class tape presentations done in Practicum Preparation II and in the supervisors' course.

Unique Components of the Training

One unique aspect of the training model described is that all participants play a number of different roles. These roles are illus-

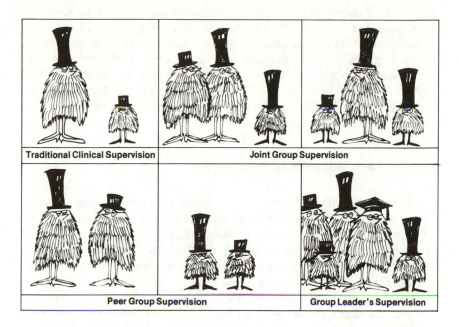

Figure 6–4. Various roles and situations used in the training model.

trated in Figure 6–4. The big owls in this figure represent supervisors, and the small owls represent students. These owls wear two different hats. In some instances, the big owls (supervisors) wear the tall (supervisory) hats. In other instances, the big owls wear the short (supervisee) hats. The same is true for the small owls (the students). In some instances, they wear the short (supervisee) hats, and in others they wear the tall (supervisor) hats. In Student-Supervisor Interactional Self-Exploratory Training, all participants are both supervisees and supervisors. In this way, the two groups develop skills in both self-exploration and the facilitation of self-exploration.

Another unique aspect of Student-Supervisor Interactional Self-Exploratory Training is the variety of supervisory encounters. These varied supervisory situations are also illustrated by the owls in Figure 6–4. Big owls (supervisors) supervise small owls (students) in traditional clinical settings. Big owls (supervisors) supervise other big owls in peer group supervision. This is also true of small owls (students). Big (supervisors) and small owls (students) meet together in joint supervisory groups. Lastly, the counseling psychologist (in the mortar board) supervises the students and supervisors in their various roles (big and small hats).

The joint supervisory training in particular deserves specific mention. Joint training undertaken in a systematic fashion has led to a clarity of expectations and a similarity of skills for those who participate in it. It allows for colleagueship and resource collaboration. The communication between supervisors and supervisees appears to be enhanced by the process. Joint training also encourages supervisors to use self-exploration to continue their growth and development as clinicians. In doing so, they model for the students self-reliant, self-actualizing professionals in an ongoing process of development.

Students' and Supervisors' Reactions

Examples taken from the student–supervisor training experiences at McGill University illustrate the issues and concerns that students and supervisors have as they learn to self-explore and assume responsibility for a mutual relationship. Specific quotations taken from training sessions or from commentary written by the students and supervisors are presented in Table 6–1.

A wide range of reactions are reflected in these commentaries. They are, indeed, thought-provoking. The reactions reveal the complexity of students' and supervisors' responses to change. They indicate the roles that these two groups of people traditionally have assumed. Furthermore, they reveal how difficult and threatening deviation from the traditional roles can be. Further study into reactions such as these is needed to increase understanding of the meaning of self-exploration for supervisors and students in Human Communication Disorders.

SUMMARY

In the first part of this chapter, the concept of self-exploration in supervision was introduced and the importance of this concept for supervisors as well as students was highlighted. The discussion was grounded in pertinent literature from the field of Human Communication Disorders and the related professional fields of Counseling Psychology, Social Work, and Psychiatry.

In the second part of the chapter, a specific training procedure used at McGill University was described. Student-Supervisor Interactional Self-Exploratory Training focuses on the development of self-exploratory abilities in students and their supervisors. The basic premise is that students and their supervisors interact in a mutual relationship. The ability to self-explore may be enhanced by this

Table 6-1.
Student and Supervisor Reactions to Interactional Self-Exploratory Training

Students		Supervisors	
• Pressure of the new demands of self-exploration	"I used to have to see clients, make lesson plans, write reports, and all that. Now I also have to watch tapes of myself, record my own behaviors, write about how I feel, guess how the client feels, think up new ideas, and tell all of that to my supervisor. It's awful!"	• Confusion over terms *direct*, *indirect*	Supervisors began by referring to a supervisory style that emphasized student self-exploration as *indirect* supervision as opposed to the previously used style of supervision, which they labeled *direct*. Group discussion led to the conclusion that perhaps a better term to use was *self-directed*. Eventually there was a consensus that self-direction and self-exploration were two different processes. Supervisors concurred that it was more helpful to think of conferences as *mutually directed*, that is, directed by both the student and the supervisor.
• Fear of confrontation	When the students were asked why they did not bring up their frustrations directly to their supervisor, one said: "Well, look, it	• Fear of confrontation	"I keep hoping that if I just forget my frustrations, they will disappear and I won't have to discuss them with the student."

Continued

Table 6-1. *(continued)*

Students		Supervisors	
• Fear of Confrontation *(continued)*	*is not that easy.* I know my grades would suffer as a consequence." "It is just that she has the upperhand. Face it— if I hurt her feelings, she will take it out on me, one way or the other.		Confrontations were never shown in the tapes presented to the joint group.
• Fear of too much control	"If I have to figure out what interests me in my tapes, I might miss some important points. I probably won't ask the right questions. My supervisor has a lot more experience than I have. She will know better what is *wrong* and what is *right* in what I did."	• Fear of lack of control	"It's beginning to sound like all our knowledge and perceptions don't mean anything. The student is deciding everything." "My students used to come like sponges to absorb all I had to say. I was the director, the leader. Now I feel like nothing."
• Difficulty in expressing the need to be less structured	It seemed to be difficult to express a need to "just talk things over." The students thought they must come to the conference with a list of points to be discussed. This sometimes served to limit the insights that a more open discussion might have produced.	• Need to find themes	"I like to figure out what is behind what my student is saying. I need to know how it relates to what we discussed last week and the week before."

• Trouble formulating alternatives	Students often said, "I didn't like how I ask for feedback. I want you to confirm that I wasn't stating my needs clearly." Rather than "I asked for feedback like this. Now I think it might have been better to say . . ." or "I would like to role-play another way to do it and see whether there are different results."	
• Concern with how to facilitate self-exploration		Often repeated phrases emerged, for instance, "What kinds of alternatives are there to how you handled the situation?"

or

"What is your interpretation of the situation?" |
• Reluctance to disclose feelings	Students never disclosed their feelings about the supervisor to the supervisor in the tapes. Written postconference notes, however, revealed a variety of feelings that had remained undisclosed during actual encounters.	
• Discomfort with positive feedback	"I want to know how you (the joint group) felt about how I received my supervisor's positive feedback. Did I appear too conceited?" Another student stated as her need that she wanted to, "figure out why I am so uncomfortable with all the positive things my supervisor is	
• Difficulty with a sense of superficiality in conferences		"My students retell the session exactly as I had just seen them perform it. I wanted to know what they *felt* and *thought* about what had happened, not just what had happened."

Continued

Table 6-1. *(continued)*

Students		Supervisors	
• Discomfort with positive feedback *(continued)*	saying to me. I keep pointing out all the negative things I did."	• Focus on understanding the students' needs	When supervisors presented tapes to other supervisors or to the joint group, they began by focusing on how well they understood the student. They searched for input from the others on how better to pick up on what the students wanted.
• Concern with making their needs known	The most frequent question asked of the joint group was "How did I ask for feedback?" The students wanted to know whether the supervisor had understood them, whether they had been able to get their needs across, whether they were able to clarify the parts that were misunderstood.	• Reaction to specificity of demands	"I'm used to doing things my own way."
		• Reaction to extra time demands	"This way of doing things takes forever."

interaction and may, in turn, enhance the interaction. Four content areas of the training were described: goal specification, tape analysis, interpersonal skills, and feedback skills. The training is experiential in format. The specific experiential protocols used for training students and supervisors in the content areas were also described.

In the final section of the chapter, remarks and concerns voiced by students and supervisors during their training were discussed. These remarks are a reflection of the reactions of the participants to the training process.

REFERENCES

American Speech–Language–Hearing Association, Committee on Clinical Supervision in Speech–Language Pathology and Audiology. (1985). Clinical supervision in speech-language pathology and audiology. A position statement. *Asha, 27*(6), 57–60.

Anderson, J. L. (1980). *Clinical supervision.* (Available from Dr. J. L. Anderson, Department of Hearing and Speech Sciences, Indiana University, Bloomington, IN)

Anderson, J. L. (1981). Training of supervisors in speech–language pathology and audiology. *Asha, 23,* 77–82.

Becker, L. B. & Silverstein, J. E. (1983, May). *SAAS: Speech act analysis system for language intervention.* Paper presented at the annual meeting of the Canadian Speech and Hearing Association, Montreal, Quebec.

Bernstein, B. L. & Lecomte, C. (1976). An integrative competency-based counselor education model. *Counselor Education and Supervision, 16,* 26–36.

Bernstein, B. L. & Lecomte, C. (1979). Self-critique technique training in a competency-based practicum. *Counselor Education and Supervision, 19,* 69–76.

Boone, D. R. & Prescott, E. E. (1972). Content and sequence analysis of speech and hearing therapy. *Asha, 14,* 58–62.

Carkhuff, R. (1969a). *Helping and human relations: A primer for lay and professional helpers — I.* New York: Holt, Rinehart & Winston.

Carkhuff, R. (1969b). *Helping and human relations: A primer for lay and professional helpers — II.* New York: Holt, Rinehart & Winston.

Cogan, M. L. (1973). *Clinical supervision.* Boston, MA: Houghton Mifflin.

Crago, M. (1980). *An adaptation of the Clezy profile for clinical analysis.* Unpublished manuscript.

Crago, M. (1982). *Clinical and supervisory skills: A series of twelve videotapes.* Montreal: McGill University Instructional Communications Center.

Crago, M. (1983, November). *Student–supervisor interactional self-exploratory training: A description and model.* Short course presented at the annual meeting of the American Speech–Language–Hearing Association, Cincinnati, OH.

Culatta, R. & Seltzer, H. (1976). Content and sequence analysis of the supervisory session. *Asha, 18,* 8–12.

Culatta, R. & Seltzer, H. (1977). Content and sequence analysis of the supervisory session: A report of clincial use. *Asha, 19,* 523–526.

Dowling, S. S. (1979). The teaching clinic: A supervisory alternative. *Asha, 21,* 646–649.

Fox, R. (1983). Contracting supervision: A goal-oriented process. *The Clinical Supervisor, 1,* 37–49.

Froehle, T. (1984). Computer-assisted feedback in counseling supervision. *Counselor Education and Supervision, 24,* 168–175.

Gizynski, M. (1978). Self-awareness of the supervisor in supervision. *Clinical Social Work Journal, 6,* 202–210.

Goldberg, D. A. (1985). Process notes, audio, and videotapes: Modes of presentation in psychotherapy training. *The Clinical Supervisor, 3,* 3–14.

Goldhammer, R. (1969). *Clinical supervision.* New York: Holt, Rinehart & Winston.

Kagan, N. (1975). *Interpersonal process recall: A method of influencing human interaction* (rev. ed.). East Lansing, MI: Mason Media.

Kaplan, N. R. & Dreyer, D. E. (1974). The effect of self-awareness training on student speech pathologist–client relationships. *Journal of Communicative Disorders, 7,* 329–342.

Littrell, J. M., Lee-Borden, N. & Lorenz, J. (1979). A developmental framework for counseling supervision. *Counselor Education and Supervision, 19,* 129–136.

Lowy, L. (1983). Social work supervision: From models toward theory. *Journal of Education for Social Work, 19,* 55–62.

McCrea, E. S. (1980). Supervisee ability to self-explore and four facilitative dimensions of supervisor behavior in individual conferences in speech–language pathology (Doctoral dissertation, Indiana University, 1980). *Dissertation Abstracts International, 41*(6), 2134-B. (University Microfilms No. 80-29, 239)

Oratio, A. R. (1977). *Supervision in speech pathology: A handbook for supervisors and clinicians.* Baltimore, MD: University Park Press.

Oratio, A. R. (1979). *Pattern recognition: A computer program for interactional analysis of intervention and training procedures in speech and hearing.* Baltimore, MD: University Park Press.

Robinson, E. E., Kurpius, D. J. & Froehle, T. C. (1979). Self-generated performance feedback in interviewing training. *Counselor Education and Supervision, 19,* 91–100.

Rogers, C. (1961). *On becoming a person.* Boston: Houghton-Mifflin.

Star, B. (1977). The effects of videotape self-image confrontation on helping perceptions. *Journal of Education for Social Work, 13,* 114–119.

Tyler, F. B., Pargament, K. I. & Gatz, M. (1983). The resource collaborator role: A model for interactions involving psychologists. *American Psychologist, 38,* 388–398.

APPENDIX A.
Supervision Contract Speech and Language Pathology

I. OBJECTIVES
  A. *Supervisor's expectations — Minimal Competencies Required* (e.g., techniques, type of patients)
    1. Involvement with four pediatric cases
      — Observation and recording of two
      — Observation and participation skills
    2. Development of observation skills
      — After observing a session, able to comment on some professional-technical skills and on some interpersonal skills
    3. Development of self-evaluation skills
      — After doing a session, able to comment on some professional-technical skills — what was effective, what was ineffective, and what was surprising
    4. Development of therapeutic skills
      — Able to use some professional-technical skills planned with or without the help of the supervisor
      — Able to convey basic interpersonal skills (e.g., interest and enthusiasm in what you are doing; empathy for the client)
    5. Development of supervision skills
      — Able to describe *your* desired supervision style
      — Able to describe other supervision styles
  B. *Student's Professional Objectives* (e.g., What are the most important things that I want to learn in this internship?)
    1. Observation of:
      a. Case history (i.e., pediatric screening if possible to schedule)
      b. Assessment
    2. Discussion of therapy planning from assessment results
  C. *Student's Personal Expectations* (e.g., self-evaluate weak and strong points; by the end of this practicum or internship, I would like to be able to . . .)
    1. Have an idea of some strengths and weaknesses

2. Have gathered from observation and from participation a list of some professional techniques for use with speech and language problems

II. ACTIVITIES
   A. *Compulsory* (e.g., department meetings)
      — Four therapy sessions observed or carried out per day
   B. *Optional* (e.g., medical rounds)
      1. Observation of (time permitting):
         a. Adult aphasia or dysarthria therapy
         b. Parent conference
         c. Case conference
         d. School visit
         e. Therapy in another discipline
      2. Familiarization with assessment and therapy materials in the department

III. METHODS
   A. *Time for Supervision* (e.g., every day for 15 minutes, or 1 hour per week)
      — At least 1 hour per day
   B. *Preparation Required for Supervision* (e.g., written resume of a case, lesson plans, tapes)
      1. Lesson plan when therapy is being carried out
      2. Brief resume of each session as required by McGill
      3. One report of a videotaped session
   C. *Style of Supervision* (e.g., direct observation, modeling)
      1. Observation by supervisor of student's sessions
      2. Use of VTR one week with report prepared for following week
      3. Attempt at indirect approach to supervision

IV. EVALUATION
   A. *Criteria for Evaluation* (e.g., number of techniques mastered, number and type of patients treated)
      1. Use of McGill evaluation form
      2. Reference to objective set
   B. *Mode of Evaluation* (e.g., self-, peer-, co-supervisors)
      1. Single supervisor and student evaluation using IV.A. 1 and 2 above
   C. *Frequency of Evaluation* (e.g., every month, 1 time per internship)
      1. Halfway through practicum
      2. Week 7

D. *Method of Appeal if Dissonant Evaluation* (e.g., co-ordinator of internship program)
   1. Discussion with Practicum Coordinator

We, _____ (supervisor) and _____ (student), agree to the conditions of the above contract, with the option that it can be modified according to circumstance as long as it is negotiated to our mutual satisfaction.

School of Human
Communication Disorders
McGill University

APPENDIX B.
Guidelines for Supervisees on Preparing for Supervision

A. Pre-Supervision
  1. Choose one case. Videotape or audiotape a clinical or supervisory session.
  2. Watching and listening to the tape, choose three segments, each about 5 minutes long:
       If you observed the session
     a. One segment in which the session was effective
     b. One segment in which the session was ineffective
     c. One segment that surprised you
       If you conducted the session
     a. One segment in which you were satisfied with your performance
     b. One segment in which you were dissatisfied with your performance
     c. One segment that surprised you
  3. For each segment, write down your impressions concerning:
       If you observed the session
     a. What you learned from this segment
     b. Your feelings/reactions during this segment, that is, the impact of the patient/client on you
     c. The effect or impact of the therapist's intervention on the patient/client
       If you conducted the session
     a. Your skill as a clinician in this segment
     b. Your feelings/reactions during this segment, that is, the impact of the patient/client on you
     c. The effect or impact of your intervention on the patient/client
  4. Choose one of the three segments to present during supervison. Write down why you have chosen this segment.

B. In-Supervision
  1. Present the case, the clinical or supervisory segment, and why you chose it.
  2. Identify the "problem" you want to deal with.

3. Define your objectives vis-à-vis this segment and this supervision session (e.g., want to determine a clear plan of what to do next time).

4. Identify your expectations of your supervisor (e.g., want confirming feedback that you handled the situation well).

5. Choose the method by which you feel you can best be helped in this supervision session (e.g., tape review, discussion, role-play).

6. Using the method chosen, go over the interview segment with the supervisor and self-evaluate a, b, and c.

7. Check your self-evaluation with your supervisor's feedback on a, b, and c.

8. Work out incongruent evaluations.

9. Explore with your supervisor alternatives for strategies whereby you can change certain behaviors or ways of interacting with patient/client.

10. Try out alternative chosen in role-play situation.

11. Self-evaluate "new behavior" and check out with supervisor's feedback.

12. Evaluate the supervision session (e.g., What did you learn? What plan of action resulted from it? Did this session respond to your needs?).

C. Post-Supervision

1. Write down what you learned from the supervision session.

2. Determine what you will do about the feedback you received.

3. Identify what you should be working on this week to improve or maintain your performance.

4. If the supervision session did not respond to your needs, identify the reasons for this (e.g., you did not present your objectives for this session clearly enough; therefore, time was spent on material that was unimportant to you).

5. Identify how you can prepare for the next session so that you get the feedback you need.

6. Set up goals for next supervision session.

APPENDIX C.
Guidelines for Supervisors on Helping a Supervisee to Analyze a Tape Segment

1. Ask the supervisee to present the case or the interviews he or she chose to discuss during the supervision session.
2. Help the supervisee to identify clearly and specifically the "problem" on which he or she would like help.
3. Help the supervisee to define his or her objectives vis-à-vis the particular case, segment of interview, and this supervision session.
4. Help the supervisee to express his or her expectations of you as supervisor, during this session (e.g., On what exactly do you want me to give you feedback?).
5. Help supervisee to choose a method by which he or she believes that he or she can best be helped (i.e., tape review, discussion, role-play). If the student is not ready to choose a method, the supervisor can suggest one. Verify whether this method is acceptable to the student.
6. Using the method chosen, go over the interview segment with the student and evaluate (without giving feedback at this point):
   a. His or her skill as a clinician
   b. His or her emotional reactions to the situation (e.g., anxious, calm)
   c. The impact of his or her interventions on the patient/client
7. Ask the supervisee to self-evaluate a, b, and c.
8. Give your feedback on a, b, and c.
9. Deal with incongruent evaluations.
10. Explore with supervisee alternatives for strategies whereby the student can change certain behaviors or ways of interacting with patient/client.
11. Try out alternative chosen in role-play situation.
12. Readjust self- and supervisor's evaluation of "new behavior."
13. Synthesis — evaluate with supervisee the supervision session (What has he or she learned? What is he or she still missing? Why were his or her needs not met in this session?).

APPENDIX D.
Guidelines on Asking for Feedback
(For both supervisors and supervisees)

1. Prepare for feedback session by first self-evaluating. Make a list of factors that impressed you positively and negatively. Ask yourself, "If I want to learn something, on what would I focus?" "What do I want to learn about?"
2. If you could ask for feedback on three factors, what would they be? They should not be questions for which you already know the answers.
3. Decide on the order of priority of factors you want feedback on. Would you like it all in one shot or item by item?
4. Describe what you want to discuss in clear, concise, and specific terms.
5. Take an active stance in thinking what you want to know about.
6. Ask for necessary clarification and elaboration from the person giving you feedback.
7. You can ask the person giving you feedback whether he or she has any other concerns to discuss.

APPENDIX E.
Guidelines on Receiving Feedback
(For both supervisors and supervisees)

1. Listen carefull to the *entire* feedback given. A good way of ensuring that you have correctly heard and that you understand the feedback is to verify your perceptions of the feedback. ". . . If I understand, what you're saying is . . ."
2. Remember that all feedback is founded on the subjective perceptions and feelings of the observer.
3. You should give as much attention to positive feedback as to critical feedback.
4. It is sometimes difficult to respond immediately to feedback. It is not expected that you respond completely and immediately to all that is said to you. However, you should position yourself generally in your immediate reaction to the feedback. Later, you can take some time and integrate this feedback and rediscuss this with the communicator.
5. It is important for the receiver to try to separate out only that which really belongs to him/her in this feedback.

APPENDIX F.
Guidelines on Giving Feedback

1. Be sure that before giving feedback, the recipient (student, peer, supervisor) has the opportunity to discuss his/her performance and feelings about it.
2. Give solicited feedback rather than focusing on what you see as being important.
3. Be sure to give feedback on the person's resources and strengths, as well as his/her limits and weaknesses.
4. Give "appropriate" feedback, that is, feedback on behavior that *can* be changed — feedback that can be used in a constructive way.
5. Give descriptive feedback based on observable facts.
6. Do not be judgmental — feedback should not focus on the other's values, beliefs, personality traits.
7. Avoid the use of clinical terms or labels.
8. Focus on the person's behavior, experience, and impact that he or she has on another (client, peer, supervisor).
9. Be clear, precise, and specific in your feedback.
10. Encourage the active exploration of the recipient of the feedback.
11. Choose your timing — immediate feedback is more productive than feedback given 2 weeks later.
12. Avoid giving too much feedback at one time.
13. Avoid giving feedback that shows off your expertise or your capacity to observe others (e.g., advanced empathy and confrontation).
14. Verify your perceptions with the recipient of your feedback (e.g., "Does that fit with the way you see things?").
    Be flexible enough to change your perceptions if need be.
15. Giving feedback implies accepting the responsibility to stay with the recipient of this feedback as long as it takes to discuss and clarify this feedback to the recipient's satisfaction (e.g., "What do you understand from my feedback — how do you feel about it?").

CHAPTER 7

Identifying Hidden Dynamics in Supervision: Four Scenarios

Vicki McCready
David Shapiro
Kathleen Kennedy

The following exchange takes place between a supervisee, who is a graduate student at a university, and her off-campus supervisor, who has worked in the local public school system for five years. "Dr. Smith" is the university supervisor who visits once a month as a liaison between the university and the public school practicum site.

Supervisee:
Marcia, when was it Dr. Smith was coming? I want to be sure he sees that voice case we've been working with.
Supervisor (apprehensively):
Next Wednesday, he'll be here all morning. What did you want to ask him?
Supervisee (defensively):
Well, I haven't formulated a list of questions or anything. I just thought he might be interested. You know, he teaches the voice disorders course at the university.
Supervisor (coldly):
Yes, I did know that.

This exchange carries with it unexpressed (and perhaps unacknowledged) feelings and thoughts that influence the quality of the communication as well as the relationship between the two people. Dynamics influencing this exchange include those arising from the relational triad of the university supervisor, the off-campus supervisor, and the student. Issues of gender, status, and academic degree as well as of power, approval, threat, and defensiveness play a role. The hidden dynamics in any interpersonal exchange are numerous and complex, and those in supervisory relationships are no exception.

This chapter uses scenarios or exchanges between supervisors and supervisees to suggest and illustrate various communicative and relational dynamics. Each scenario includes the actual dialogue and the supervisor's and supervisee's feelings and thoughts during the dialogue. The scenarios are divided into two sets, one set illustrating participant and setting dimensions of the supervisory process, and one set illustrating instruction and evaluation dimensions. The presentation of the two scenarios in each set is preceded by a discussion of relevant literature and is followed by a partial replay of the same situation in order to suggest and illustrate different interpersonal dynamics.

PARTICIPANT AND SETTING DIMENSIONS OF THE SUPERVISORY PROCESS

Because of the nature of institutions in which supervision takes place, particular experiences occur that can influence the supervisory process and relationship. Furthermore, cultural values, attitudes, and needs of the individual participants in the process can affect supervisory interactions. Information about the participants and the various settings in which the process takes place should contribute to an understanding of the interpersonal dynamics that may be operating.

Characteristics of Individual Participants

Various studies provide information about supervisees and supervisors.

Supervisees

Students in Human Communication Disorders are typically white, female, and pursuing a bachelor's degree in speech–language pathology (Council of Graduate Programs in Communication Sciences and Disorders, 1985). As Table 7–1 indicates, the majority of students pursuing careers in Human Communication Disorders at the under-

TABLE 7-1.
Degrees Awarded in the Discipline in 1983–1984

	Bachelor's (%)	Master's (SLP) (%)	Master's (A) (%)	Master's (SP SCI) (%)	Doctoral (SLP) (%)	Doctoral (A) (%)	Doctoral (SP SCI) (%)
Female	93.3	95.1	83.5	95.2	73.8	40	37.5
Male	6.7	4.9	16.5	4.8	26.2	60	62.5

Adapted from Council of Graduate Programs in Communication Sciences and Disorders (1985, September). *1984–85 national survey.*
(Available from National Survey, P.O. Box 1903, University, AL 35486)

SLP = speech-language pathology; A = audiology; SP = speech science graduate level and at the master's level in speech–language pathology, audiology, and speech science, as well as at the doctoral level in speech–language pathology, are women. More men than women are pursuing audiology and speech science at the doctoral level.

Some investigators have studied the perceived supervisory needs and expectations of student clinicians at different levels of clinical training. Using a descriptive survey design to analyze the responses of experienced and inexperienced clinicians, Larson (1982) found that experienced student clinicians expected to state opinions, design strategies, and apply their ideas. They also expected their supervisors to be supportive, to attend to what they were saying, and to listen to their professional problems. Inexperienced student clinicians also expected to be actively involved but, in addition, expected their supervisors to tell them the weaknesses in their clinical behavior. The strongest needs of both groups were to receive support from supervisors and be allowed to express their opinions. Larson concluded that affective needs are continuous throughout training, whereas the need for technical supervision decreases as students gain experience.

Dowling and Wittkopp (1982) and Myers (1980) also found that supervisees had different needs as a function of their different levels of experience. For example, Dowling and Wittkopp found that beginning students expressed a need for direct suggestions for diagnosis and treatment of clients, whereas more advanced students wanted increased clinical responsibility and reduced supervisory input. In Myers' study, the technical needs of clinicians appeared to decrease in importance with increased training. Affective needs, however, appeared to be continuous throughout training.

Supervisors

As the data in Table 7–2 from the Council of Graduate Programs in Communication Sciences and Disorders (1985) indicate, most clinical supervisors both on- and off-campus are women. Furthermore, women constitute most of the faculty on-campus supported by soft money and most of the full-time and part-time positions at the master's degree level. At the doctoral level, most of the faculty in full-time as well as part-time positions are men. As reported by Fein (1984), data collected by ASHA surveys in 1982–1983 indicate that 83 percent of ASHA members who engaged in clinical supervision as their primary activity were women, 17 percent were men.

Although little else is known about supervisors as a group, a study by Schubert and Aitchison (1975) noted that the majority of

Table 7-2.
Some Characteristics of Clinical Supervisors and Faculty in HCD* in 1984–1985

	Supervisors Off-Campus (%)	Supervisors On-Campus (%)	Faculty On Soft Money (%)	Faculty In Full-Time Positions (%)	Faculty In Part-Time Positions (%)
Female	84	76	13.0 (Master's) 4.5 (Doctoral)	81.1 (Master's) 34.9 (Doctoral)	86 (Master's) 40 (Doctoral)
Male	16	24	8.6 (Master's) 3.4 (Doctoral)	18.9 (Master's) 65.1 (Doctoral)	14 (Master's) 60 (Doctoral)

Adapted from Council of Graduate Programs in Communication Sciences and Disorders (1985, September). *1984–85 national survey.* (Available from National Survey, P.O. Box 1903, University, AL 35486).

*Human Communication Disorders

university supervisors were women between the ages of 26 and 32 years, employed full-time in 9- to 10-month positions.

Rassi (1985) has suggested that two types of supervisors exist, primary and secondary. She defines the secondary supervisor as a faculty member with a doctorate who is hired for the purpose of teaching and research, and is given clinical supervision as a secondary assignment. The primary supervisor, on the other hand, is a person with a master's degree who identifies supervision as the primary responsibility.

Setting

Because students in speech–language pathology and audiology are in a variety of practica settings as they fulfill ASHA certification requirements, it is important to understand the characteristics of those settings that may influence supervisory interactions.

In the university setting, personnel include both clinical and academic faculty who differ in their academic degrees and the tenured or nontenured status of their positions. Clinical supervisors, often in positions of fixed length, may comment that they have limited opportunity to participate in departmental decisions and feel of low-status and distanced from other faculty.

Another consideration for supervisors in university settings is that of multiple and, at times, conflicting responsibilities. University supervisors, like all ASHA members, must adhere to the ASHA Code of Ethics (ASHA, 1984), which notes that the needs of the client are paramount. Furthermore, supervisors have a responsibility to address the university's commitment to student learning. These two obligations can, at times, be in compatible.

Clinical programs at most universities use the public school as a practicum setting. Noticeable differences exist between university-based supervision and public school–based supervision. Supervisors in the public school are generally unpaid for their supervisory services. In addition, they must balance the needs of their own clients in a typically large caseload with the needs of the student clinician. Another difference between settings pointed out by Dowling (1981) is that unlike the university supervisor who observes the supervisee sporadically, the public school supervisor typically interacts daily and intensely with the supervisee.

Public school supervisors frequently interact not only with their clients and the student supervisee but also with a university liaison supervisor, a person whose function may not be understood fully by either the student or the school supervisor. The student clinician may feel caught in the middle, wondering whether he or she should follow the directives of the university liaison supervisor, the public school supervisor, and/or the supervisor's supervisor (e.g., the school principal or the head of the special services staff).

Other off-campus practicum sites include hospitals and clinics. Supervisors in these sites are generally unpaid for their supervisory work and often spend considerable time in supervision (Ehrlich, Merten, Sweetman & Arnold, 1983). Because of various funding policies, staff members functioning as supervisors need to be present most of the time when services are provided. In the opinion of Ehrlich and colleagues (1983), the setting of the hospital clinic does not allow the luxury of a "hands-off" approach to supervision, which would allow students to experiment and make mistakes.

Another issue in some off-campus clinic and hospital sites is that of financial pressure on staff to treat a minimum number of patients per week. Furthermore, patients in hospitals tend to move in and out of therapy quickly, thus presenting the staff with large numbers of people in short periods of time. Lastly, although university liaisons should bridge the gap between the university and the off-campus site, the off-campus supervisor can feel isolated in his or her supervisory work and not receive needed support and guidance.

In summary, the characteristics of supervisors and supervisees and the settings in which they practice can affect specific interactions between individual supervisors and their supervisees, as the following scenarios show.

Illustrations of Participant and Setting Dimensions of the Supervisory Process

The scenarios in this section suggest and illustrate dynamics associated with participant and setting factors. These dynamics relate to roles and settings and to issues involving status and gender. After a brief discussion of the hidden dynamics in each scenario, a partial replay of the situation reveals what can happen when a new set of dynamics operates.

Scenario 1: The Triad of University Supervisor, Student Supervisee, and Off-Campus Supervisor

Scenario 1 offers a second look at the same exchange presented in the introduction to this chapter, but this time the thoughts and feelings that both supervisor and supervisee have during the exchange are revealed.

The situation in this scenario involves the student supervisee, Susan, and her off-campus supervisor, Marcia Brown, who has a master's degree and works in the local public school system. Michael, who has a voice disorder, is their client, and Herman Smith is the liaison supervisor from the university who visits once a month. The setting for the exchange is Marcia's therapy room in the public school. Dynamics illustrated are territoriality, threat, status, and gender.

SCENARIO 1.
The Triad of University Supervisor, Student Supervisee, and Off-Campus Supervisor

The Actual Exchange	Supervisor's Internal Thoughts	Supervisee's Internal Thoughts
Supervisee: Marcia, when was it Dr. Smith was coming?* I want to be sure he sees that voice case we've been working with.	Boy, do I feel inadequate here. My supervisee needs to consult with the university supervisor about a child on *my* caseload. Don't they teach students tact anymore? Does Marcia think I don't know what I'm doing? Doesn't she know that my first responsibility here is to my caseload?!	The child reminds me so much of a case Dr. Smith presented to our voice class. I bet he might have some ideas about what we might try.
Supervisor (apprehensively): Next Wednesday he'll be here all morning. What did you want to ask him?	Maybe, I can find out what it is she hasn't been able to get from me.	Wonder what's going on with Marcia. She sounds d at me. What have I done wrong?
Supervisee (defensively): Well, I haven't formulated a list of questions or anything. I just thought he might be interested. You know he teaches the voice disorders course at the university.	I don't think I believe her reason here. And I'm feeling threatened. Susan and Dr. Smith might both think I don't know what I'm doing. I wonder if I'd feel differently if Dr. Smith were a woman.	Actually, I thought he could help us. Michael has continued to abuse his voice for months now. For some reason, I'm scared to tell Marcia this.

The Actual Exchange	Supervisor's Internal Thoughts	Supervisee's Internal Thoughts
Supervisor (coldly): Yes, I did know that.	And so what if he teaches the voice course? I've been working with our school district's voice program for 3 years now and feel like I have "real world" experience that has been invaluable. So *why* am I feeling so upset and threatened here?	What is going on here?
Supervisee: Is it O.K. with you? I mean, that Dr. Smith sees Michael?	Well, now I feel better, back in control. She's asking me for permission.	Maybe, I should have asked her this in the first place. Oh dear! Sometimes I feel caught between two supervisors. Yuk! It's hard enough to please one supervisor, let alone two!
Supervisor: Sure, but I don't know what he'll be able to tell us that we don't already know.	Susan needs to know that I am knowledgeable just Like Dr. Smith. I don't have a "Dr." in front of my name, but I do know what I've done with this particular case and I feel good about it. I'm feeling unappreciated by Susan. Not only do I not get paid for my supervision, I don't get appreciation either. And I do tire of her talk about her experiences at the university.	I'm feeling really confused now. Yes, he can see Michael but what good can he do? I think I'd better pull out of this. It's too late in the semester for me to risk making Marcia mad. And jeopardize my "A."

(continued)

Scenario 1 *(continued)*

The Actual Exchange	Supervisor's Internal Thoughts	Supervisee's Internal Thoughts
Supervisee: Well, I doubt if I'll be able to change Michael's therapy time from PM to AM anyway . . . no big deal. You're probably right too, we already know why Michael's not changing.	Funny, I don't feel any better hearing Susan say this. In fact, I think I feel worse and I'm not sure why.	Wonder if she'll believe this. Gee, I sure hope Marcia's not mad at me anymore.

*The manner in which supervisees address their supervisors is a complicated issue and may vary according to clinical training programs and individuals. The scenarios in this chapter were written with this variance in mind.

The involvement of a university supervisor in the work of a student clinician and off-campus supervisor can complicate the interpersonal dynamics of the supervisory process. In this situation, Marcia feels threatened by Susan's wanting to consult the university supervisor about a child on their caseload. In addition, she feels as though her territory is being invaded and her authority and expertise doubted. She is aware that the university supervisor has a doctorate and is addressed as "Dr." and wonders whether his gender or his academic degree makes a difference either to her or her student. She also thinks she is in a vulnerable, low-status postion, both because of her degree and her work setting. Although she views her setting as more like the real world than the university clinic, she and her student might be ascribing more power to the university and the expertise of its teachers than to the experience and expertise of the public school clinician.

Replay of Scenario 1: The Triad of University Supervisor, Student Supervisee, and Off-Campus Supervisor

The replay of Scenario 1 illustrated the effect a different set of dynamics can have on the same situation. The dynamics illustrated include self-awareness, openness, collegiality, and sharing.

Replay of Scenario 1.
The Triad of University Supervisor, Student Supervisee, and Off-Campus Supervisor

The Actual Exchange	Supervisor's Internal Thoughts	Supervisee's Internal Thoughts
Supervisee: Marcia, when was it Dr. Smith was coming? I want to be sure he sees that voice case we've been working with.	I could feel very threatened here. After all, I've been out of school a few years, away from the university environment, and I do tend to feel low-status when *Dr. Smith* is mentioned. Think I need to do some checking out with Susan.	The child reminds me so much of a case Dr. Smith presented to our voice class. I bet he might have some ideas about what more we might try.
Supervisor (openly, curiously): Next Wednesday morning. What do you have in mind?		
Supervisee: Well, Dr. Smith told us in class one time about a very similar case, and I was wondering whether he would have any ideas about how we could help Michael more.	Now, I'm starting to feel unappreciated and unacknowledged.	
Supervisor: He might. Susan — you know, you and I may come up with some more ideas if we did some more talking.	I don't feel like telling her my feelings just yet — I'm not sure if I will.	Oops, I bet I should have talked to Marcia about Michael first. I think I was afraid of bothering her.

(continued)

Replay of Scenario 1 *(continued)*

The Actual Exchange	Supervisor's Internal thoughts	Supervisee's Internal Thoughts
Supervisee: That would be great. I haven't asked you before cause I know how busy you are, and I'm always afraid I'm bothering you too much.	I had no idea she may be hesitant to ask me questions! I sure am busy with my caseload, but I would have discussed Michael with her.	
Supervisor: Oh! And here I was feeling a little defensive because you wanted to consult with Dr. Smith, and you hadn't shared any of your concerns about Michael with me. I was not feeling very valued.		WOW! I had no idea my supervisor might feel defensive or not valued. Gee, she sounds human, like me with my self-doubts.
Supervisee: Gee, I sure didn't mean to imply that.		

In this replay, the overall tone permeating the exchange is quite different from that in the original scenario. Although Marcia still feels threatened and unappreciated, she is aware of her tendency to have these feelings and tries to remain open to her supervisee's intent. She proceeds with an attitude of collegiality toward Susan, as exemplified by her tone and her use of the pronoun "we." Susan feels free to share some of her feelings openly and nondefensively. The exchange closes with Marcia, too, sharing feelings.

Scenario 2: A Triad of A Male Supervisor,
Female Supervisor, and Male Client

Scenario 2 depicts a situation involving a 30-year-old male super visor, Jack Jones; a 16-year-old male client, Rick; and a 20-year-old supervisee, Mary. The setting for the first part of the exchange is the hallway of the university clinic; the second part of the exchange takes place during a supervisory conference in Jack's office. Dynamics illustrated are sexual attraction, undifferentiated feelings, and authoritativeness.

SCENARIO 2.
A Triad of a Male Supervisor, Female Supervisee, and Male Client

The Actual Exchange	Supervisor's Internal Thoughts	Supervisee's Internal Thoughts
Supervisor: Mary, there's something I need to talk to you about. Would you mind making an appointment to meet with me?	They never told me how to handle this in my supervisory training! I've got to get Mary, who is in her early 20s, to understand why Rick, her 16-year-old client who stutters, won't go into the therapy room without me. I think Rick finds Mary attractive and doesn't know how to handle it.	I can't stand it when a professor says this. It's so hard to wait to find out what you've done wrong! And Dr. Jones seemed so nervous and serious when he asked to see me. I've been doing all my work; I get all my lesson plans in on time.
Supervisee: O.K. Is something wrong?		
Supervisor: I just need to talk to you about your client, Rick.	And here I am Mary's male supervisor, understanding how Rick could find her attractive; yet I need to be counseling her about the situation. I guess, in part, I'm uncomfortable because I, too, find Mary attractive.	Oh boy, do I dread that talk. I don't know why Rick won't go into therapy with me alone. I feel like I haven't been standing on my own two feet.

(continued)

SCENARIO 2 *(continued)*

The Actual Exchange	Supervisor's Internal Thoughts	Supervisee's Internal Thoughts
Supervisor (later in conference): Mary, why do you think Rick refused to work with you alone?	I just haven't known how to approach this whole situation.	Sounds like Dr. Jones knows something I don't.
Supervisee: Gosh, I don't know, I've sure felt terrible though that you have to be in there with me all this time.	Surely, Mary must be aware of how others may perceive her, including her attractiveness.	I'm getting more and more anxious. I wish he would just get to the point.
Supervisor: Have you ever stopped to think how you might be coming across to him?	She's looking startled and confused. How naive can she be? Do I have to spell it all out?	What is he getting at? I've never treated any of my clients that differently.
Supervisee (defensively): I don't do anything differently with him that I do with other clients.	Rick told me he just wasn't used to being alone with "girls," but I could tell he was attracted to Mary immediately, as was I.	I feel like I'm on the witness stand being interrogated. I've got to get to the bottom of this.

It may happen that male supervisors, who supervise primarily female students, will find one of those students attractive; in addition, male clients may also find their student clinicians sexually attractive. Although not portrayed in this particular scenario, other situations involving attraction may exist; for example, female students may feel attracted to their male supervisors, or female supervisors may feel attracted to their male students. In this scenario, what Jack has not realized is that just as sexual attraction may be interfering with the clinician–client relationship, it is also interfering with the supervisor–supervisee relationship. Jack, who himself finds Mary attractive, is not fully aware of his own feelings in this situation and interacts with Mary in an authoritative, accusatory manner.

The kind of exchange Jack and Mary have in their supervisory conference is consistent with findings in the literature that supervisors tend to share few personal thoughts and rarely help students expand their expressions of feelings (Pickering, 1984). Just as in the first scenario, the supervisor and supervisee focus more on the client than on any interpersonal concerns in the supervisory relationship.

Replay of Scenario 2: A Triad of a Male Supervisor,
Female Supervisee, and Male Client

The replay of Scenario 2 illustrates the effect of the supervisor's changing his attitude and language, sharing his own thoughts, and tuning in to the supervisee's feelings. Dynamics in this replay include respect, reflection, sharing, and self-awareness.

Replay of Scenario 2.
A Triad of a Male Supervisor, Female Supervisee, and Male Client

The Actual Exchange	Supervisor's Internal Thoughts	Supervisee's Internal Thoughts
Supervisor: Mary, I'd like to talk with you about how things are going with Rick. Do you have some time now?	I'm feeling very nervous about this whole situation, and I want to handle it in a way that doesn't blame Mary but does alert her to the effect she may be having on Rick.	I'm glad Dr. Jones wants to know how things are going. I've really needed to talk to him.
Supervisee: Sure.		
Supervisor: Let's talk about how we're each perceiving the situation of his not wanting to be in the therapy room alone with you. What do you make of it?		I like the way Dr. Jones seems to respect my opinion, even in this awful situation.
Supervisee: Gosh, I don't know. I sure feel terrible that you have to be in there with me all the time.		

(continued)

Replay of Scenario 2 *(continued)*

The Actual Exchange	Supervisor's Internal Thoughts	Supervisee's Internal Thoughts
Supervisor: Like you should be handling this more on your own?		
Supervisee: Yeah, I feel like I haven't been standing on my own two feet . . . has Rick told you why he won't be with me alone?		
Supervisor: He has said that he wasn't used to being alone with girls. I'm wondering if he may be feeling attracted to you now and is scared to have those feelings.	Gee, as I say those words I wonder if I've been scared to have those same feelings for Mary, myself, as if it's wrong for me, her supervisor, to have them. I need to remember that I don't have to disclose them and that Rick, the client, may not necessarily be experiencing the same feelings as I.	
Supervisee: Wow! Do you really think so? I'm so embarrassed that I didn't even think of this. I guess I was seeing Rick just as a fluency client and was forgetting he's also a 16-year-old boy.		Even though I'm embarrassed, I'm so glad Dr. Jones is alerting me to what may be happening.

In this replay, Jack approaches Mary in a respectful manner, asking if *she* has time to meet and asking what *her* perceptions of the situation are. When Mary shares her feelings, Jack listens and makes a reflective statement. He shares some of his thoughts and has an insight into his own feelings and assumptions. He is aware that he does not have to share all these feelings with Mary and thinks that too much self-disclosing could create additional problems.

Additional Illustrations of Participant and Setting Dimensions

Other scenarios could illustrate the part that participant and setting aspects might play in the supervisory relationship. Imagine the following situations in which characteristics such as gender, age, status, and family background may be playing their parts:

• A supervisor and supervisee, working in an open collegial relationship, seek additional advice on their adult fluency client from the faculty member who teaches the fluency courses. The faculty member strongly recommends that they both sit in on her course to review the content that she thinks they should have known before working with a fluency client. The supervisor is left feeling incompetent and embarrassed, and the supervisee does not know how to react.

• The department chairperson interrupts a supervisory conference to remind the supervisor of a special faculty meeting that has been called. Although the supervisor had just scheduled an important conference with her supervisees at that same time, she tells the chairperson, in front of her supervisee, "no problem, I'll be there. I just have to cancel a conference"; the supervisee concludes that supervision and therapy are less important than faculty business.

• A 30-year-old female supervisor who has been supervising for only two years is working with a 37-year-old female supervisee who has returned to school after teaching for several years and raising her own two children. The supervisor views this nontraditional student as she would any other student — as a younger person who needs to be told about "professional" behavior. The supervisee feels resentful and wants more personal and professional respect, and the supervisor feels insecure and threatened.

• A 20-year-old female undergraduate is being supervised by a 50-year-old male supervisor who has a directive, authoritative manner. The young student, who has many unresolved issues with her father, frequently defers to this supervisor, who, in turn, fosters the student's dependence.

This section of the chapter has dealt with various participant and setting dimensions of the supervisory process that may affect the interpersonal dynamics between supervisor and supervisee. Issues relating to the characteristics of each participant such as gender, status, and needs, as well as those issues unique to particular settings, were illustrated in two different scenarios as well as in additional descriptions of situations.

INSTRUCTION AND EVALUATION DIMENSIONS OF THE SUPERVISORY PROCESS

Of the myriad of clinical teaching dimensions of the supervisory process, two can be singled out for particular attention: instruction and evaluation. The supervision literature has included information on both these processes. Such information should contribute to an understanding of the personal dynamics that may be operating in a supervisory relationship.

Instruction

The supervisory conference is "at the heart of clinical teaching" (Pickering, 1982, p. 38) and is considered by Anderson (1980) to be the most important supervisory activity. What do supervisors think they teach in the conference and in the process? According to ASHA's 1985 Position Statement on Clinical Supervision in Speech–Language Pathology and Audiology, "effective clinical teaching involves, in a fundamental way, the development of self-analysis, self-evaluation, and problem-solving skills on the part of the individual being supervised" (ASHA, 1985, p. 57). The tasks of clinical teaching involve helping the supervisee set goals and objectives and develop and refine observation, assessment, and management skills. In addition, supervisors have the task of helping students resolve interpersonal issues in clinical relationships with their clients and in supervisory relationships with their supervisors.

Numerous research studies in supervision have investigated the content of supervisory conferences and have found that a primary focus is on instruction. Schubert and Nelson's (1976) analysis of the verbal behaviors of supervisors and supervisees indicated that the largest percentage of behaviors used in conferences were generated more by supervisors than by supervisees. Supervisors provided opinions, suggestions, and factual information. Although questions of reliability and validity have been raised about their analysis system

(Dowling, Sbaschnig & Williams, 1982), Culatta and Seltzer (1976) found that supervisors did most of the talking and provided most of the teaching strategies in conferences. Even when given a chance to change their behaviors over time, supervisors continued to do most of the problem-solving and directing in conferences (Culatta & Seltzer, 1977). Using a different system of analysis, Roberts and Smith (1982) came up with similar findings. In their study, supervisors dominated the conference by structuring and soliciting responses, whereas supervisees took a more passive role, following the lead of supervisors, responding to their questions, and participating less. Supervisors and supervisees were consistent in maintaining these behaviors over time. Although most of the research has found that supervisory conferences focus primarily on instruction, at least one study (Pickering, 1984) indicated that conferences were multipurposed and included some emphasis on interpersonal concerns involving clients.

Self-analysis is often a major consideration in discussions of clinical teaching (Anderson, 1981; Crago, Chapter 6 of this volume; Oratio, 1977). Shattuck-Hansen, Kennedy, and Laikko (1985) spoke to this issue in their recent study of supervisory conferences and suggested that if instructing students in learning to self-analyze and problem-solve is among the primary goals of supervision, supervisors may want to examine the role they take in conferences to determine whether, in fact, they are meeting this goal.

Evaluation

The evaluation component of clinical teaching involves giving feedback to supervisees about their performance in different supervisory and clinical skill areas. It also includes assisting the supervisee in developing skills of self-evalution (ASHA, 1985).

The evaluation systems that have been reported in the literature demonstrate that supervisors expect students to develop and change in the areas of technical and interpersonal skills. A widely used system is the Wisconsin Procedure for Appraisal of Clinical Competence (W-PACC) (Shriberg et al., 1975). It evaluates students at different skill levels according to their clinical and academic experience. On the 38-item form, student clinicians are rated according to the type and amount of sypervision they need in order to be effective. A student with more clinical hours would be expected to need less supervisory direction and to demonstrate more independence than a beginning student with few or no clinical hours.

Another evaluation system, this one developed at the University of Texas at Dallas, is the Competency Based Evaluation System

(Lougeay-Mottinger, Harris, Perlstein-Kaplan & Felicetti, 1984). It divides students into four ability levels from Entry to Advanced, based on clinical and academic experience, and uses different rating definitions from"good" to "not evident" for the four ability levels. Just as with the W-PACC, students can see how their performance is expected to change from a basic to a more advanced level with increasing experience.

Several studies have indicated that both supervisors and supervisees have particular attitudes about the grading and feedback components of supervision. For example, Russell and Halfond (1985) found that six graduate student supervisees and six supervisors viewed clinical grades as necessary, inevitable, ultimately useful, and anxiety producing. The supervisees saw grades as a measure of their worth, and the supervisors described grades as the most difficult aspect of clinical teaching. In their study of 52 students' perceptions of the supervisory process, Wollman and Conover (1979) found that the possibility of a poor therapy grade influenced the students' behaviors with supervisors and with peers in the clinic. In Dowling and Wittkopp's (1982) study of 191 undergraduate and graduate student clinicians, students indicated that they liked written evaluative feedback following an observation, positive and negative feedback about their clinical behavior, supervisory encouragement to use self-evaluation techniques, and formal evaluation and discussion of their clinical behavior. They did not like clinical experiences in which they were given no feedback.

Another area of concern to both supervisees and supervisors is the way in which feedback is given (Dowling, 1981; Pickering, 1981; Smith, 1981). Smith (1981) advised supervisors to examine carefully the function, focus, and form of feedback given during supervisory interactions. She recommended that supervisors strive to function as colleagues to their supervisees by providing feedback in objective ways so that during a final evaluation, the relationship and objective basis for discussion have been established. In her discussion about providing feedback in constructive ways, Pickering (1981) described the experiences of threat and defensiveness that all humans share, as well as the climates that tend to evoke defensiveness, for example, the climates of negative judgment, attempted control, and absolutism. Dowling (1981) emphasized that evaluation should be minimal and carefully presented in a supportive manner. She suggested that the supervisees evaluate themselves prior to the supervisor's provision of feedback.

The evaluation aspect of clinical teaching is a complex one that can include giving evaluative and nonevaluative feedback and grades to supervisees for individual therapy sessions and overall clinical performance. An important aspect to the entire evaluation dimension of supervision is the interpersonal climate in which feedback and evaluations are given.

Illustrations of Instruction and Evaluation
Dimensions of the Supervisory Process

The two scenarios in this section suggest and illustrate some of the numerous interpersonal dynamics associated with instructing and evaluating and with being instructed and being evaluated. Discussions and replays follow each scenario.

Scenario 3: The Instructional Process

Scenario 3, which takes place in an audiology supervisor's office, involves Kay Frank, an audiology supervisor who has a master's degree and is in a soft-money position in the university clinic, and her supervisee Teri, an audiology student nearing the end of her graduate school training. They are conferring on a Friday, prior to a hearing evaluation that they have together on Monday. The dynamics include control, power, and rescue.

Scenario 3.
The Instructional Process

The Actual Exchange	Supervisor's Internal Thoughts	Supervisee's Internal Thoughts
Supervisor: Teri, I think your plan for the diagnostic evaluation on Monday looks generally fine. I do have a few suggestions, of course. But don't worry, I'll be there with you for the interview and most of the testing.	I feel good about how I'm always there for my supervisees. Unlike tenured faculty who supervise but can never be found, I'm accessible. And I do like being needed, too. Students are so inexperienced, and our clients need the best expertise they can get.	Geez! Here I am, a fourth semester graduate student with almost 300 clock hours of supervised audiology practicum, and I can't be trusted to do any evaluation on my own. Why won't my supervisor give me more room to grow and show my independence? Does she think I'm not capable?

(continued)

Scenario 3 *(continued)*

The Actual Exchange	Supervisor's Internal Thoughts	Supervisee's Internal Thoughts
Supervisee: Oh, that's O.K. You can join me if you like, but you don't really need to.	What is this? Our students now tell us when and when not to supervise? I feel unappreciated enough by the other faculty and now by my own student too!	The truth of the matter is that I don't want her to join me whether she wants to or not. But, I just couldn't say it; I'm afraid I'll hurt her feelings. And, she does look offended.
Supervisor (hurt tone): Well, if you feel that way about it, I guess you can try. I do need to ensure that the client gets the best service we can give her.	I want her to acknowledge me more and admit she needs me. How can I get her to do this?	Obviously, she's hurt anyway. And now, she's implying I'm selfish and not thinking of the client. Oh boy!
Supervisee: Gee, I'm sorry. I don't want to shortchange the client, of course . . . come on in and join us, really.	Well, that's more like it. She knows I have more to offer the client. I feel better now, more in control and needed.	Oh well, I don't want to upset her anymore. I'm about to graduate and get out of here anyway. I can't wait to be on my own.
Supervisor: We'll see. I may need to.		

Kay, the supervisor in this scenario, does not perceive that her advanced student has made progress; instead, she treats the student like a beginning clinician in need of a considerable amount of guidance, explanation, and demonstration. Teri, the supervisee, does not have the same kinds of technical supervisory needs she had when she was a less-experienced audiology student (Larson, 1982; Myers, 1980). Kay, although diligent and well intentioned, is influenced by her needs to be needed and to be in control. She does not see Teri's need for independence. Rather than focusing some of the conference interaction on Teri's feelings and reactions, Kay directs attention to the client's needs. Kay feels herself in a low-status, unappreciated position and relies on her supervisees to give her the power and authority she lacks among her colleagues. She has fallen into what Hornyak (1980) calls "the Rescue Game" (p. 86). If she can rescue her supervisees by giving the right answers, she can continue to feel needed and knowledgeable. Teri feels powerless and deprived of independence.

Replay of Scenario 3: The Instructional Process

The replay of Scenario 3 illustrates a different set of dynamics at work in the instructional process: collegiality and sharing.

Replay of Scenario 3.
The Instructional Process

The Actual Exchange	Supervisor's Internal Thoughts	Supervisee's Internal Thoughts
Supervisor: Teri, we have a diagnostic together on Monday. How are you feeling about it?	I need to remember that Teri is one of my more experienced supervisees, who may not need my help on this evaluation. I'll do some checking with her before jumping in to help.	I'm so glad Kay is checking with me on this one. I want to tell her how capable I'm feeling now.
Supervisee; Fine. I've done several diagnostics for preschoolers with suspected conductive hearing losses. I think I've chosen the appropriate test battery, and I've given all the tests before.	Boy, that's hard for me to hear ... Teri has outgrown me. Why do I have such trouble letting go?	
Supervisor: You know you're sounding more and more independent. How does that feel?	I want to give her credit for becoming more independent.	Boy, is it nice to hear that word — independent! Hoorah!

(continued)

Replay of Scenario 3 *(continued)*

The Actual Exchange	Supervisor's Internal Thoughts	Supervisee's Internal Thoughts
Supervisee: Great! I never thought I'd see the day.	I think I also need to share where I'm at with Teri. If I don't, I may not be able to keep supporting her.	
Supervisor: You know, as hard as it is for me to admit, I sometimes have trouble letting go of students.	Whew! I'm glad I said it, but I do wonder how Teri will see me now.	
Supervisee: Gosh Kay, I never considered what it must be like for you. I always see you as the competent supervisor you are.	That's interesting. Maybe by hiding some of my feelings and needs, I've presented myself as a professional who doesn't have them.	I guess I forgot that Kay's human too; she always seems together, so on top of everything.
Supervisor: Gee, it's nice to hear that from you Teri!	I forget that I not only can give to my students but also can receive openly from them ... I wish my own colleagues and I could do the same ...	I wish I had thought to give Kay more appreciation this semester. As a student, I get so caught up in my own stresses, I make the assumption that our teachers don't need our support.

In this replay, the supervisor begins to foster and support her supervisee's independence. The supervisory relationship becomes more collegial, and both participants show their respect for one another. They also begin to share their feelings and needs with one another, and thereby learn more about themselves. Kay, the supervisor, is beginning to realize the contrast between her supervisory relationships and her faculty relationships.

Scenario 4: The Evaluation Process

Scenario 4 is a mid-term supervisory conference in which Phyllis Lee, the supervisor, and Sara, the supervisee in her first practicum experience, need to discuss their evaluation of Sara's clinical skills. Responsibility, blame, defensiveness, and control are the dynamics illustrated.

SCENARIO 4.
The Evaluation Process

The Actual Exchange	Supervisor's Internal Thoughts	Supervisee's Internal Thoughts
Supervisor: Well, Sara, it's time to discuss your performance in practicum at this mid-term point.	Here we go again. . . the marginal student. Sara's neither failing nor doing poorly enough to be counseled out of the program, and here's a client not getting the treatment she could be getting. I've just given out an evaluation weighted more with weaknesses than strengths, and I know that by not giving much praise, I'm not facilitating good learning conditions. I sure will be glad when this conference is over!	Boy, do I dread this meeting. Things just haven't been clicking for me this semester, and I am feeling so pressured to perform the way Ms. Lee wants me to. All I'm getting is criticism, and I just don't know if I can keep going. And now a "C" at the mid-term! I've never gotten a "C" in any of my classes before.
Supervisee: Uh-huh.	She sure sounds discouraged and depressed. And I'd sure like to help her feel better. I feel like the bearer of only bad news.	I just know I'll cry, and I don't want to do that in front of Ms. Lee.

(continued)

The Actual Exchange	Supervisor's Internal Thoughts	Supervisee's Internal Thoughts
Supervisor: As you know, I've some concerns about some of your skills. So, my evaluation and grade should not have come as a surprise to you. Did they?	She looks distraught and surprised. How could she be surprised? We've been working on her areas of weakness for weeks now.	You better believe a "C" was a surprise! Guess I better not admit my surprise. I should have known, just like Ms. Lee is saying ... but, I have been doing better.
Supervisee: Well, I guess not ... I did think I had been improving recently ... I just don't know what you want.	Boy, do I hate to hear that last line! She doesn't know what I want, as if what I want is different from the principles of good teaching. She's putting it all on me.	Sure would be nice to hear something positive RIGHT NOW!
Supervisor: I thought I had been making clear to you some changes I think might help your client.	All those extra hours I've put in with this student — sure would be nice to get even a "thank you."	What about ME and what I think? I can't stand this pressure to change.
Supervisee: I tried so hard in that last session with Ellen. It took me hours to cut out all those pictures, and she loved them! And all I got was criticism about how I wasn't praising her enough, I wasn't firm enough with her.	Students can sure get into that headset of time and effort equal quality work with the client! I guess I could have praised her for those pictures ... well, we could talk all day about that one session ...	Maybe she'll give me a little bit of praise and credit if I tell her how hard I worked on that last session.

(continued)

SCENARIO 4 *(continued)*

The Actual Exchange	Supervisor's Internal Thoughts	Supervisee's Internal Thoughts
Supervisor: Let's see if we can stay on track here and just talk right now about your evaluation.	I'm not liking the way I'm handling all this. I've been feeling defensive and that's made me tight and tense ... defensive and unappreciated.	No, she won't even acknowledge that I did do something well! Shall I keep feeling angry or just give up?

In this scenario, the well-meaning university supervisor feels caught between client and student and takes responsibility for the progress of each. Aware that she has to grade and give feedback to a marginal student who has more weaknesses than strengths, Phyllis does not know how to conduct the conference. She chooses an authoritative, controlling stance, placing blame on Sara for her reaction and putting pressure on her to change. Both Phyllis and Sara engage in mutual attack and defense until Phyllis changes the topic abruptly, regaining her control and authority.

This scenario and the dynamics in it raise an important issue that supervisors face regularly as part of the supervisory process, that of giving grades and feedback to supervisees. Supervisors may or may not have enough training in the supervisory process or enough knowledge about interpersonal dynamics to create an atmosphere in which students can receive feedback in nondefensive ways and can deal with their feelings.

Replay of Scenario 4: The Evaluation Process

In the following replay of Scenario 4, the supervisor, by changing some of her own behaviors, alters the overall interaction. Dynamics illustrated are self-awareness, reassurance, sharing, and clarification.

In the replay, Phyllis, the supervisor, listens to the supervisee's feelings while staying aware of her own. Sara, the supervisee, believes that she has been heard and feels freer to share some of her thoughts. Phyllis continues to promote a trusting atmosphere by being appropriately empathic, positive, and reassuring. In addition, she shares some of her own previously concealed feelings and attempts to clarify her expectations. In this interaction, both supervisor and supervisee are more self-aware and self-sharing than in their previous interaction.

REPLAY OF SCENARIO 4.
The Evaluation Process

The Actual Exchange	Supervisor's Internal Thoughts	Supervisee's Internal Thoughts
Supervisor: Well, Sara, it's time to discuss your performance in practicum at this mid-term point.	This situation with the marginal student is always hard for me...I tend to feel caught in the middle between student and client, wanting them both to change. I start feeling anxious and tense, and I lose sight of the student. I want to stay aware of my tendency here and tune into Sara more.	Boy, do I dread this meeting. Things just haven't been clicking for me this semester, and I am feeling so pressured to perform the way Ms. Lee wants me to. All I'm getting is criticism, and I just don't know if I can keep going. And now a "C" at the mid-term! I've never gotten a "C" in any of my classes before.
Supervisee: Uh-huh.	She sure sounds discouraged and depressed.	I just know I'll cry, and I don't want to do that in front of Ms. Lee.
Supervisor: You look upset.		She's right! I am upset.
Supervisee: I am! (crying)...Oh! I didn't want to cry in front of you...	I'm so glad she's letting herself cry. She sure looked like she wanted to hold on to those tears.	As much as I wanted to hide my feelings from her, I'm glad she noticed. And I know I'll feel some relief after I cry.
Supervisor: It's O.K. (offering some Kleenex and sitting with Sara quietly)	At least I can comfort her some.	

The Actual Exchange	Supervisor's Internal Thoughts	Supervisee's Internal Thoughts
Supervisee: It's just that I've never gotten a "C" before in any of my classes. I really thought I had been doing better recently (crying).	Sounds like she needs some positive feedback from me. I know I haven't been giving much.	Now I've blown it. She knows I'm grade conscious! Oh well — what do I have to lose at this point?!
Supervisor: Well, you have been trying and working a lot harder recently. I could tell you put a lot more thought into that last session with Ellen.		
Supervisee: It's good to hear I've been doing something right.		Whew! Maybe there's hope after all!
Supervisor: Yes — I know that helps. . . I guess you haven't been hearing much positive feedback from me over the last 2 weeks.	When there is so much negative, I do find it much harder to find something positive to say.	WOW! It's so nice to hear a supervisor talk about what she hasn't been doing! I might as well find out if Ms. Lee has been trying to tell me that I need to drop out of practicum. With all the negative feedback I've been getting, I sure have wondered.
Supervisee: No, I haven't! I was starting to wonder if I should change fields.	She is certainly not a candidate for me to counsel out. Wonder if I've been sending that message?	

(continued)

REPLAY OF SCENARIO 4 *(continued)*

The Actual Exchange	Superviser's Internal Thoughts	Supervisee's Internal Thoughts
Supervisor: Oh dear! I haven't meant to send that message.		
Supervisee: Maybe I just haven't known what you wanted.	Hmm — I could get very defensive and angry over that statement. But, she sounds sincere, and I don't think it would be helpful at this point for me to launch into a discussion of how that statement pushes a button in me . . . she may be right too. In all my worry about the client's making progress, I may not have been clear with Sara.	
Supervisor: Well, Maybe I haven't been clear enough about my expectations. Sometimes I start feeling so responsible for you and your client, I lose sight of how I'm coming across to you.		WOW again! I'm not feeling so alone in this whole process. If my supervisor's so willing to look at herself, I can surely do the same.

Additional Illustrations of Instruction and Evaluation Dimensions

Other exchanges between a supervisor and supervisee suggest interpersonal dynamics related to clinical teaching dimensions of the supervisory process. Imagine the following:

• A supervisor decides to intervene in what she determines is an unproductive session. She demonstrates a modification in the activity that works for the client but leaves the supervisee feeling incompetent and inferior. The supervisor feels pleased with her demonstration and considers it an effective instructional technique.

• A supervisor and parent are observing a session in which the child has just thrown a temper tantrum. Although the supervisee is attempting to work things out with the child, the parent wants the situation handled differently and is pressuring the supervisor to intervene. The supervisor feels caught in the middle — she wants to give her supervisee more time, yet she also wants to please the parent.

• A supervisor has asked his supervisee to sign up for a conference and is feeling impatient and angry that the supervisee has not done so. The supervisee, feeling incompetent, has been presenting himself as a cool, competent clinician. He is avoiding a supervisory conference because he fears being found out.

• A speech–language pathologist working in a hospital is supervising a staff member's Clinical Fellowship Year. Although the new clinician came with good recommendations as well as a good academic record, she has been making inappropriate diagnostic decisions and handing paperwork in late. The supervisor feels angry and confused about the discrepancy between the supervisee's record and performance, and uncomfortable about confronting the supervisee, especially since the two are close in age.

This last section of the chapter has focused on clinical teaching aspects of the supervisory process, specifically the instructional and evaluation dimensions, and how they influence interpersonal communication between supervisor and supervisee. In the scenarios and descriptions that illustrated these dimensions, concerns about grading and giving feedback to students and about teaching students with different levels of training were presented.

CONCLUSION AND CONSIDERATIONS

It has been the premise of this chapter that increased recognition and understanding of interpersonal dynamics can enhance the supervisory process. Four scenarios illustrated some of the dynamics that both research and experience suggest may be operative. Actual research on the process is needed to identify the specific interpersonal dynamics that are present. In addition, research on supervisors' characteristics, needs, and expectations as well as research on the characteristics of different practicum settings would be helpful in furthering the understanding of supervision.

In addition to research, there are ways in which supervisors can increase their understanding of the interpersonal dynamics affecting the supervisory process. A support group for supervisors, for example, might be a helpful forum in which supervisors could share and discuss some of the issues identified in this chapter, such as status and gender issues. Supervisors wanting to gain self-awareness and to understand the complexity of communication may benefit from individual counseling, further study of interpersonal communication, or instruction in counseling skills.

In order to study interpersonal skills in supervisory interactions, supervisors could study transcriptions of verbal and nonverbal interactions made from audio- or videotapes. Analysis of an exchange written in the way presented in this chapter and perhaps facilitated by use of one of the interaction analysis systems might reveal some previously unrecognized dynamics.

REFERENCES

American Speech–Language–Hearing Association. (1984). Code of ethics. *Asha, 26*(1), 70–71.

American Speech–Language–Hearing Association, Committee on Supervision in Speech–Language Pathology and Audiology. (1985). Clinical supervision in speech–language pathology and audiology. A position statement. *Asha, 27*(6), 57–60.

Anderson, J. L. (Ed.) (1980). *Proceedings Conference on training in the supervisory process in speech–language pathology and audiology.* Bloomington, IN: Indiana University.

Anderson, J. L. (1981). Training of supervisors in speech–language pathology and audiology. *Asha, 23*(2), 77–82.

Council of Graduate Programs in Communication Sciences and Disorders. (1985, September). *1984–85 national survey.* (Available from National Survey, P.O. Box 1903, University, AL 35486).

Culatta, R. & Seltzer, H. (1976). Content and sequence analysis of the supervisory session. *Asha, 18,* 8–12.

Culatta, R. & Seltzer, H. (1977). Content and sequence analysis of the supervisory session: A report of clinical use. *Asha, 19,* 523–526.

Dowling, S. (1981). Supervising student teachers: How to provide non-threatening feedback. *Journal of Childhood Communication Disorders, 5,* 153–156.

Dowling, S., Sbaschnig, K. V. & Williams, C. J. (1982). Culatta and Seltzer content and sequence analysis of the supervisory session: Question of reliability and validity. *Journal of Communication Disorders, 15,* 353–362.

Dowling, S. & Wittkopp, J. (1982). Students' perceived supervisory needs. *Journal of Communication Disorders, 15,* 319–328.

Ehrlich, C. H., Merten, K., Sweetman, R. H. & Arnold, C. (1983). Training issues: Graduate student externship. *Asha, 25*(12), 25–28.

Fein, D. J. (1984). Vive la difference??? *Asha, 26*(1), 35.

Hornyak, A. J. (1980). The rescue game and the speech–language pathologist. *Asha, 22*, 86–89.

Larson, L. (1982). Perceived supervisory needs and expectations of experienced vs. inexperienced student clinicians. (Doctoral dissertation, Indiana University, 1981). *Dissertation Abstracts International, 42*, 4758B.

Lougeay-Mottinger, J., Harris, M. R., Perlstein-Kaplan, K. E. & Felicetti, T. (1984). UTD competency-based evaluation system. *Asha, 26*(11), 39–43.

Myers, F. (1980). Clinician needs in the practicum setting. *SUPERvision, 4,*(2), 7.

Oratio, A. R. (1977). *Supervision in speech pathology: A handbook for supervisors and clinicians.* Baltimore, MD: University Park Press.

Pickering, M. (1981). Supervising student teachers: How to provide non-threatening feedback. *Journal of Childhood Communication Disorders, 5,* 150–153.

Pickering, M. (1982). *Supervisory manual in communication disorders.* Orono, ME: University of Maine, Department of Speech Communication.

Pickering, M. (1984). Interpersonal communication in speech–language pathology supervisory conferences: A qualitative study. *Journal of Speech and Hearing Disorders, 49,* 189–195.

Rassi, J. A. (1985). Clinical supervision in a university setting. Competencies, qualifications, training: Audiology. In J. E. Bernthal (Ed.), *Proceedings of the Sixth Annual Conference on Graduate Education* (pp. 26–32). Lincoln, NE: University of Nebraska, Council of Graduate Programs in Communication Sciences and Disorders.

Roberts, J. E. & Smith, K. J. (1982). Supervisor–supervisee role differences and consistency of behavior in supervisory conferences. *Journal of Speech and Hearing Research, 25,* 428–434.

Russell, L. H. & Halfond, M. M. (1985, November). *An expanded view of the evaluative component of clinical supervision.* Paper presented at the annual meeting of the American Speech–Language–Hearing Association, Washington, DC.

Schubert, G. W. & Aitchison, C. J. (1975). A profile of clinical supervisors in college and university speech and hearing training programs. *Asha, 17,* 440–447.

Schubert, G. W. & Nelson, J. A. (1976). An analysis of verbal behaviors occurring in speech pathology supervisory conferences. *Journal of the National Student Speech and Hearing Association, 4,* 17–26.

Shattuck-Hansen, D., Kennedy, K. B. & Laikko, P. A. (1985). Verbal interaction patterns in supervisory conferences: A preliminary investigation. *Journal of the National Student Speech–Language–Hearing Association, 13,* 20–35.

Shriberg, L. D., Filley, F. S., Hayes, D. M., Kwiatkowski, J., Schatz, J. A., Simmons, K. M. & Smith, M. E. (1975). The Wisconsin procedure for appraisal of clinical competence (W-PACC): Model and data. *Asha, 17,* 158–165.

Smith, K. J. (1981). Supervising student teachers: How to provide non-threatening feedback. *Journal of Childhood Communication Disorders, 5,* 147–150.

Wollman, I. L. & Conover, H. B. (1979). The student clinician's perception of the supervisory process. *Ohio Journal of Speech and Hearing, 14,* 192–201.

CHAPTER 8

Interpersonal Communication and the Supervisory Process: A Search for Ariadne's Thread

Marisue Pickering

As I have pondered the complexities of supervisory interactions and the supervisory process, the image of a maze has often come to mind, and I have felt akin to those Greek mythological figures who tried to find their way through the Labyrinth. And, like Theseus, I have needed an Ariadne's thread to lead me through. I have needed help in making sense out of my interactions with students and my students' interactions with clients. The "threads," that have helped me the most have come from two bodies of literature: Humanistic-existential thought and Interpersonal Communication. In this chapter, I present what I consider critical themes from these two literatures before focusing on aspects of interpersonal communication and the supervisory process. Then after a brief look at empathy and associated behavioral skills, I conclude the chapter with a set of basic assumptions about interpersonal communication and supervision.

HUMANISTIC-EXISTENTIAL THOUGHT

Humanistic-existential thought has been an influence not only on my professional work but also on that of others in our field, for example, Caracciolo, Rigrodsky, and Morrison (1978a), Luterman

(1979), Murphy (1982), and Oratio (1977). In addition, its impact has been significant on scholars in other helping professions as well as in interpersonal communication. Exemplars include Sieburg (1985) in family therapy, Collier (1982) in counseling, Kübler-Ross (1969) in thanatology, Garvin and Kennedy (1986) in nursing, and Stewart (1986) in interpersonal communication.

My first exposure to the humanistic-existential literature was literary, specifically the works of existentialists such as Sartre and Camus. In addition, Martin Buber, Victor Frankl, Abraham Maslow, and Pierre Teilhard de Chardin were early (and enduring) influences. Later, I discovered such people as Charlotte Buhler, R. D. Laing, and Elizabeth Campbell. At the risk of over simplifying the numerous and complex themes in humanistic-existential thought, I will briefly discuss only six major points. These particular points have guided my understanding of what the supervisory relationship is — and can be — about.

The Validity of Individual Perception

Many philosophers and psychologists have stressed that what a person perceives and how he or she interprets reality is valid for that person. Buber (1965, 1966) developed this idea in depth, stressing the importance of recognizing the uniqueness of others and of affirming and confirming them as individual beings. Maslow's (1966) work helped validate the importance of the psychological study of people as individuals, with their own unique experiences and realities. Acknowledging the validity of individual perception means putting aside one's own frame of reference in order to hear the other. It also means honoring the affective, poetic, and intuitive side of human beings.

The Possiblity of Dialogue or Mutuality

Dialogue is based on the self being in relation to others and on the belief that individuals can and do move toward hearing and understanding each other. Buber's (1958, 1965, 1966) writings developed the essense of dialogue from both theological and philosophical perspectives. Dialogue has to do with collaborating, facilitating, and negotiating and is in contrast to imposing on the other or denying the other's perceptions. Dialogue depends on lack of pretense, lack of defensiveness, and lack of reservation about the worth of the other.

The Potential of Individual Choice

Even when choice of behaviors is extremely constrained, psychologists such as Frankl (1963) have suggested that individuals have a choice of attitudes. Basing much of his work on his concentration camp experiences, Frankl believes that the last and, at the same time, the most basic human freedom is the ability to choose one's attitude in a given set of circumstances. In communication, the potential and possibility of choice can be seen in options available for responding as well as in attitudinal options. We can and do choose one set of behaviors, one communicative style over the other.

The Relationship of Behavior and Intent

Counselors such as Pedersen (1982), as well as philosophers such as Searle (1983), have worked with the concept of intentionality in relation to interpersonal communication. Understanding intent suggests taking responsibility for choices and identifying one's basic stance or goal toward the other. In communication, intent has to do with what a person hopes to bring about as a result of the communicative interaction. Behaviors are linked to intent, even when intent is unknown, vague, or ambiguous. A heightened awareness of intent can lead to an increase in behavioral options. Such increased "response repertoire" is a goal both in interpersonal communication (Smith & Williamson, 1985) and in counseling (Ivey & Galvin, 1983).

The Importance of Human Growth and Transformation

The belief that people "grow" implies that human beings can move beyond particular constraints. Individuals can and do change. Buhler (1971) argued for a psychology that reflected the importance and reality of human growth and evolution. For her, homeostatis was not a guiding principle. Humanistic psychologists talk often about the human's ability to evolve and to create meaning. As Campbell (1984) stated, "given a nourishing environment, humans have the potential to develop as a [sic] self-determining, self-actualizing, self-transcending healthy persons" (p. 16). The work of Jesuit paleontologist Teilhard de Chardin (1959) also contributes to viewing life from a growth or evolutionary perspective.

The Insistence on Being Holistic

Humanistic psychology stresses the importance of approaching individuals holistically. This means viewing people systemically and relationally. Campbell (1984) noted that humanistic psychologists have developed skills for working with family systems as well as with organizational systems. Buber and Laing are among those who stress the existential nature of people *in relationship:* "For the inmost growth of the self is not accomplished . . . in man's relation to himself, but in the relation between the one and the other" (Buber, 1965, p. 71). Further, "That is to say, the ground of the being of all beings is the relation between them. This relationship is the 'is,' the being of all things" (Laing, 1967, p. 23).

In sum, humanistic-existential thought provides an ethical base for relationships, a set of secular values that complement those of many Western theologies, and a theoretical foundation for research and practice in helping relationships. Nevertheless, thought-provoking criticisms do exist. For critiques of humanistic psychology in particular, see, for example, Campbell (1984) and Greenspan (1983).

INTERPERSONAL COMMUNICATION

The second major set of readings that has helped me make sense out of supervisory interactions is from the field of Interpersonal Communication.

Although from the beginning of my work as a clinician and later as a supervisor, I realized that "interpersonal communication" was a critical dimension of the process, it was some time before I learned that it was also an academic field of study and research. Writings in the field of Interpersonal Communication range from discussions of theoretical issues to presentations of particular skills and competencies. The discussions that I have found particularly relevant to the supervisory process pertain to (1) models of communication, and (2) particular axioms or principles of communication.

Models of Interpersonal Communication

Models probably are an attempt to explain and shape practice. Thus, they offer a simplified overview of a complex process. I find communication models helpful in informing my understanding of supervisor–student interactions as well as student–client interactions.

According to interpersonal scholars Smith and Williamson (1985), three different models account for the differing scholarly views of the nature of interpersonal communication. The first, the action model, focuses primarily on the behavior of only one person in the interaction. This view of interpersonal communication is illustrated in research studies that examine an individual's particular communication style. In Human Communication Disorders, reports that focus on communicator style characteristics (e.g., Sorenson, 1983) or on clinical interaction skills (e.g., Shriberg, et al., 1975) are suggestive of this model of communication. An advantage of applying this model is that research is relatively simple to design and carry out, and much can be learned about particular skills or competencies used in interactions. A disadvantage is that only one partner in the dyad is studied, and the interaction and the relationship not at all.

The second model, referred to as the interaction model, is an information or message-centered model. This model acknowledges the importance of each person in the dyad and stresses the mutual or reciprocal influence of each one on the other. The importance of "receiving, decoding, interpreting, and acting upon messages" is basic to the interaction model (Smith & Williamson, 1985, p. 10). This model is illustrated in research that examines what people say to each other. In Human Communication Disorders, systems that analyze information exchange, whether through simple or complex means, appear to view communication through such a model. Such systems include those reported by Boone and Prescott (1972), Oratio (1979a, 1979b), and Smith and Anderson (1982). An advantage to this view of communication is that it looks at interactions and patterns of interaction *over time*. Furthermore, with the advent of computer-assisted analyses, large amounts of data can be studied. A problem with this model is that information exchange and message sequencing are not the totality of human interaction; thus, an over-simplified understanding of dyadic communication can result.

The third model, referred to as the transactional model (Smith & Williamson, 1985), is concerned with the nature of the dyadic relationship as well as with patterns of information exchange. The *relational* dimension of messages, not simply their content dimension, is investigated. The perspectives and roles of the two individuals who are mutually perceiving and adapting to each other are considered. This model focuses on the *meaning* that evolves from the interaction and thus is considered to be meaning-centered rather than message-centered (interaction model) or speaker-centered (action model). Studies reflecting this complex understanding of communication might focus

on information exchange, in order for aspects of the relationship —
not just the messages — to be understood. Or the focus might be on
the meaning that the relationship has for its participants, and the
data collection might include use of journals or interviews. The
analysis is often of the relationship rather than the message or the
speaker (Wilmot, 1979).

In Human Communication Disorders, a research effort that
reflects this view of interpersonal communication is Pickering and
McCready's (1983) analysis of supervisors' journals. This study
focused on the meaning of the supervisory relationship for the supervisors. Still, only one person in the dyad was studied; students' views
were not considered.

An advantage to the transactional model of communication is
that it acknowledges the complexity of individuals-in-relationship. A
major problem is that traditional research methodologies are often
inappropriate, and alternative methods have to be developed — not
always a viable option.

An additional discussion of models of communication and their
applications in clinical work in Human Communication Disorders
can be found in an earlier work (Pickering, 1985).

Selected Axioms or Principles of Interpersonal Communication

In any field of study, there are certain basic axioms undergirding
theory, research, and practice; the field of Interpersonal Communication
is no exception. Three axioms in particular have been helpful in enhancing my understanding of supervisory and clinical interactions.

Communication is Transactional

This axiom is the basis for the transactional model of communication. It suggests that communication occurs *between,* not *in,*
individuals. Together and mutually, members of a dyad (or other social
unit) create what happens. Application of this principle to supervision means that an in-depth analysis of a supervisory or a clinical
session would include a focus on (1) communicative behaviors and
roles of *each* person, (2) the meaning that the communication appears
to have for each person, (3) the interpretations made by each person,
(4) patterns of communicative behaviors over time, and (5) relational
changes over time. The focus would be on the dyadic partners and
their relationship, not simply on one person or on the messages exchanged.

Point of View Determines Meaning

This axiom suggests that in a communicative transaction, any action can be seen as the cause *or* the effect, depending on the participant's perspective. This axiom further suggests that each individual will recall the situation differently and may define or label the situation differently. An example of the first instance is the experience of recalling that the other person began or "caused" a conflict and that the self is the blameless victim. An example of the second instance is the experience of a child defining a clinical situation as calling for a protest (perhaps by hitting), and the adult defining the situation as calling for a need to control the child. The child thus might consider the hitting to be appropriate action, whereas the clinician defines it as uncooperative, noncompliant, or immature behavior. When analyzing clinical or supervisory sessions, designating one event a cause and another event an effect is probably less helpful and less important than analyzing the sequence and meaning of the communicative patterns. Further discussion of this idea can be found in Chapter 5.

Individuals Function in a Relational System

This axiom acknowledges that individuals do not exist alone, but live and function within a social network of meaning. Thus, the relational system itself is important to consider. Some of the most important work on this perspective has been done by the Palo Alto School of communication theorists, including Bateson (1972), Watzlawick and Weakland (1977), and Wilder (1979). In the field of Human Communication Disorders, applications of a relational systems perspective have been made in children's language disorders (Hubbell, 1981), language assessment and intervention (Conant & Budoff, 1984), family involvements (Andrews & Andrews, 1984), and clinical and supervisory processes (Pickering & VanRheenen, 1985). This axiom corresponds with the two others just discussed in its stress on looking at communication in terms of relations rather than in terms of entities. Thus, communicative phenomena are explained not only in terms of their components but also in terms of relationships between and among components. Systems are approached more appropriately as wholes with interacting parts than as constituent parts adding up to a whole.

In addition to these three axioms, others that are important to consider and that I have discussed elsewhere (Pickering, 1985) are as follows:

1. Communication is a process, not a thing.
2. Communication is circular, not linear.
3. Communication involves the total personality.
4. Communication is complex.
5. In a transaction, an individual cannot *not* communicate.
6. Meaning, ideas, and information are conveyed through a variety of message systems, of which oral language is only one.
7. Messages have more than one level of meaning.
8. Transactions involve individuals at multiple levels of perspective.
9. The self is created and maintained through interpersonal transactions.

These 12 axioms should not be reified. As knowledge about the nature and function of interpersonal communication increases, it is likely that the degree of sophistication about its axioms and principles will also increase.

THE SUPERVISORY PROCESS AND INTERPERSONAL COMMUNICATION

There is no way to disassociate interpersonal communication from the supervisory process. It is one of the crucial dimensions of supervision, and various scholars have provided additional skeins of Adriadne's thread in their efforts to understand it. In this section, many of these efforts will be mentioned briefly before three broad competencies germane to the analysis of interpersonal communication are discussed.

A Review of Concerns and Efforts

Practicum supervisors in Human Communication Disorders have had at least three areas of concern in relation to interpersonal communication. The first has to do with themselves and enhancing their own knowledge, attitudes, and skills. Much of the supervisory literature relevant to interpersonal aspects has focused on what supervisors could do to make themselves better communicators.

Specific emphasis has been, for example, on managing conflict (Farmer, 1986a), on understanding defensiveness and learning confrontational skills (Ward, Antwine, Hillard, Covington & Barker, 1984), on developing self-exploratory skills (Crago, 1983), on learning strategies of verbal and nonverbal pacing (Farmer, 1986b), on providing nonthreatening feedback (Pickering, 1981), on applying concepts from humanistic-existential thought (Pickering, 1977), or on identifying particular interpersonal skills (Schmitt & Gibbs, 1984–85).

A second area of concern has focused on providing appropriate interpersonal and facilitative conditions for student growth and development. Representative work in this area includes that by Caracciolo, Rigrodsky, and Morrison (1978a, 1978b), McCrea (1980), Oratio (1977), and Ward and Webster (1965a, 1965b).

Parts of this chapter as well as Chapters 6 and 7 focus, either directly or indirectly, on these two inseparable areas of concern.

A third area of concern has to do with helping students discuss, analyze, and improve their interpersonal attitudes and skills in relation to clients. Although the profession at large has not made the kind of commitment to the development of interpersonal skills that it has to the development of other skills (e.g., no required coursework in interpersonal communication for the CCC or for ESB accreditation), individual practitioners and researchers have seen the interpersonal dimension as a vital component of the clinical endeavor, for example, Emerick and Hood (1974), Hagler (1985), Hubbell (1981), Klevans, Volz, Fiore, and Love (1980–81), and Murphy (1982).

In order to help student–clinicians develop their interpersonal attitudes and skills, those engaged in clinical teaching have reported two major types of efforts: skill training procedures and conference-based pedagogical strategies.

Skill Training Procedure

Only a few individuals have attempted to develop or enhance students' knowledge about interpersonal communication or their interpersonal skills.

Kaplan and Dreyer (1974) reported an experimental study in which students were trained in self-awareness skills, and Rosenthal (1977) reported a peer group therapy experience for student–clinicians in beginning practicum. Moore (1979) reported an effort to develop interpersonal skills simultaneously in stuttering clients and their student clinicians. Another dual approach to training was reported by Crago (1983), this one in relation to skills of self-exploration and involving student–clinicians and supervisors. Crago further explicates her model in Chapter 6.

Major efforts in training students in specific interpersonal skills have been reported by Volz, Klevans, Norton, and Putens (1978). Their findings indicated "that speech–language pathology undergraduates . . . typically use few verbal responses considered helpful in the development of an effective client–clinician relationship" (pp. 539, 540).

Following this initial research, additional programs — influenced by models in counseling — were developed to help undergraduates learn appropriate verbal skills (Klevans, Volz & Friedman, 1981). Research on these programs suggested that "length of training may be a crucial variable as students appear to need considerable time and practice to master the complex skills necessary for interpersonal effectiveness" (p. 208). In addition to length of training, another significant issue surfaced: Does the counseling literature offer appropriate models for training the interpersonal skills of individuals in our profession? Furthermore, in another discussion, Klevans and Volz (1978) asked: "If interpersonal skills can be taught, when is the best time to teach them?" (p. 63). Such concerns have yet to receive concentrated attention.

Another effort at interpersonal communication skill training has been reported by Hagler (1985) in his work with undergraduate practicum students. He concentrated on "assertion-based communication skills" (p. 3) and used extensive role-playing. Although Hagler's results are preliminary and need further confirmation, he has provided an additional attempt to speak to this "neglected area of student training" (p. 5).

The development of skill training procedures — at least as reported in the professional literature — is still in its infancy in speech-language pathology and audiology. Nevertheless, the need to help students enhance their understanding of interpersonal communication remains. An approach of a different sort is summarized in the following section.

Pedagogical Strategies

Working from the assumption that clinical supervisors in Human Communication Disorders are likely to be the individuals most involved in helping students enhance their knowledge and skills of interpersonal communication, a colleague and I (Pickering & VanRheenen, 1984–85) focused on the supervisory conference (and process) as a context for teaching interpersonal communication. We suggested three types of teaching:

1. Didactic Teaching: Supervisor as Educator, Teacher
2. Skill Training: Supervisor as Trainer, Shaper
3. Indirect Teaching: Supervisor as Role Model

In didactic teaching, supervisors supply the students with knowledge and information about interpersonal communication, just as they would about specific aspects of, for example, learning theory. This can be done through discussion, assigned readings, or transcript analysis. The major point is that the conference can be used as a place for supervisors to educate students about ideas and concepts central to interpersonal communication.

A second way to use the conference for teaching interpersonal communication is through actual skill training. VanRheenen and I noted the importance of being behavioral and task oriented when shaping interpersonal skills and suggested three strategies: direct instruction on the target skill, role-playing the skill, and self-evaluation of the new skill. Thus, just as the conference can be used to shape planning and instructional skills, it can be used to shape interpersonal skills.

The third way that the supervisory conference — and the supervisory process as a whole — can be used for teaching interpersonal skills is through role-modeling. For example, through the use of empathic behaviors or through discussions with students about communication intent, supervisors serve as role models. Conversely, if a supervisor considers a focus on interpersonal issues, including the expression and discussion of affect, to be inappropriate, that too can become a model for the student–clinician. As we stated, "Indeed, supervisors are role-models and might want to probe their own behaviors in relation to what it is they are implicitly and explicitly expecting of students" (p. 7).

Although not subjected to rigorous investigation, these ideas are practical and manageable as pedagogical strategies for the clinical teaching of interpersonal communication constructs and skills.

Competencies Germane to Communication Analysis

One of my concerns is how — within the context of the supervisory conference — to help student–clinicians analyze interpersonal issues involving their clients. Little is known about the depth and breadth to which students in Human Communication Disorders use the supervisory process for this purpose. One study (Pickering, 1984) reported that within supervisory conferences, students identified more interpersonal issues pertaining to clients than did the supervisors. This suggests a commitment on the part of those students to sorting through interpersonal issues. The subsequent discourse was primarily solution oriented, rather than discussion oriented, and no consistent, systematic approach to communicative analysis was evident. This suggests that an in-depth understanding of communication analysis was missing in students as well as in supervisors.

Enhanced effectiveness in communication analysis can occur in several ways. For example, helpful analysis systems or protocols are available in our literature, the interpersonal literature, and the helping professions literature. In addition, I believe there are competencies that can enrich those supervisory discussions that focus on making sense out of clinical interactions. Three such competencies — all derived from the transactional model of communication — are presented here.

Putting the Self in the System

The idea that human interaction has systemic qualities has been discussed by numerous communication scholars and has been developed in some detail vis-à-vis clinical and supervisory relationships (Pickering & VanRheenen, 1985). Thinking of the systemic nature of human interaction means thinking in terms of interrelated parts. It means realizing that the helper and the helpee are part of a system and are mutually influencing and shaping one another.

Traditionally, supervisors and students may not have put themselves into the system when describing and analyzing interpersonal encounters. For example, in a study of conference interactions (Pickering, 1984), I found that, "When students discussed interpersonal issues involving clients, they did so not as problems in the interactions between themselves and the clients but as problems *in* the clients" (p. 192).

In order for supervisors and students to appreciate the nature of dyadic interaction, they must realize that *they* are a part of a system. When students analyze clinical interactions, they need to include an analysis of *their* actions, patterns, and experiences. They need to act on the knowledge that the other person is not the primary unit of analysis — they both are. Or better yet, their system, their relationship, is that which calls for description and analysis.

Identifying Patterns Over Time

Looking at communicative patterns in relationships is a crucial aspect of communication analysis. Hocker and Wilmot (1985), in discussing patterns of conflict in relationships, noted that patterns and regularities occur not only in verbal interactions, but also in the rules that are followed and in the dynamics of the particular system. Certain patterns are probably generic to all dyadic relationships, and other patterns are specific to each relationship. Wilmot (1979) noted that when studying dyadic communication, which is what the student–clinician is doing when discussing a clinical encounter with the supervisor, the *pattern* of interaction, or the series of patterns, is an appropriate unit of analysis (p. 13).

In Human Communication Disorders, several reports (e.g., Pickering & McCready, 1983; Roberts & Smith, 1982; Smith & Anderson, 1982) indicate that patterns of verbal interaction can be seen within the supervisory process. Even though it can be assumed that patterns exist in all interactions, it is difficult for individuals to identify and analyze their own interactional patterns, especially if the interaction is at all conflictual. Because of this difficulty, a third party can offer assistance. Such assistance is, of course, one of the major contributions a supervisor can make when the student–clinician discusses clinical interactions. For this to happen, however, supervisors, as well as students, need to develop abilities in pattern analysis.

Understanding Relational Issues

As noted earlier, communication scholars have stressed the importance of viewing communication as relational, that is, as something that happens *between* rather than *in* people. Within this conceptual framework, authors such as Bennis, Schein, Steele & Berlew (1980) have addressed the purpose of the relationship for the dyadic partners. Thus, if a client has in mind a different purpose for the clinical relationship than does the student–clinician, problems may result. Any analysis of clinical interaction will need to be cognizant of this relational issue.

Another relational issue concerns the roles assumed by the dyadic partners (Wilmot, 1979). For example, a role may be based on personal attitudes (I need help) or on professional knowledge (I am a competent clinician). Understanding roles in this context has to do with understanding social identities; the term does not imply that a person is acting in a false manner. In analyzing clinical transactions within the supervisory process, it may be necessary to examine whether or not the client and the clinician are assuming mutually compatible roles.

A third issue addresses content talk and relational talk. Discourse contains both content and relational messages. Thus, the statement from a student–clinician to a child, "Don't do that," attempts to control a behavior on the level of content. It also carries with it the message that the student–clinician has the right and the authority to exert that type of influence, and, of course, the client may not always agree. Realizing that messages have a relational as well as a content level and bringing that knowledge to bear during interactional analyses can enhance the depth of analysis.

A somewhat different approach to understanding relational issues has been presented by Farmer (1985–86). In his discussion of relational development in supervisory conferences, he focused on assumptions about change, learning, and communication styles. Farmer's work, directed toward supervisors, is also relevant to student–clinicians as they consider relational development in clinical sessions.

Understanding that relational issues exist and are explicated through communicative transactions is a crucial competence for both students and supervisors.

Applying these three competencies when analyzing interactions will take effort. Supervisors and student–clinicians will need to continue their work as partners in the supervisory process in order to develop the appropriate sophistication and expertise necessary both to apply the transactional model to understanding communication and to use the supervisory process to analyze interpersonal dimensions of the clinical process.

SUPERVISION AND EMPATHIC COMMUNICATION

Certainly there are numerous helpful ways to respond to students, but one way has to do with accepting or confirming them as individuals. Often the term *empathy* is used in this regard, and supervisors (and clinicians) are often urged to be empathic. Use of this term seems to me to be similar to the use of the term *rapport* when I was an undergraduate. We were told "to establish rapport" but without a lot of clarity about what actually to do. Thus, this section focuses briefly on one additional part of the supervisory maze: confirming or empathic communication.

Empathy is a complex phenomenon that has drawn the interest of writers in numerous fields in addition to ours, for example, Interpersonal Communication, Education, Counseling, Psychology, and Psychotherapy. According to one writer (Hill, 1982), empathy "originated with the German word *einfuhlung* which translates as the 'process of feeling into' " (p. 83). It has been seen as an essential component for counseling relationships (Egan, 1975; Rogers, 1958) as well as a facilitative condition for relationships in general (Hill, 1982).

At the minimum, empathy is the ability to let students know that the obvious meaning of their words has been understood. A higher level of empathic understanding involves the ability to go beyond words and put together cues found in tone, gesture, and context, and then to respond to a student's fuller meaning. Empathy means hearing and seeing how the students' messages reflect their perspectives, rather than modifying their messages to agree with the supervisor's perspective. Empathy thus means listening as a *receiver* rather than as a critic and responding in accepting rather than in evaluative ways.

Operationally defining a construct as multifaceted as empathy runs the risk of oversimplification and reification. Furthermore, discussing behavioral skills without a concomitant discussion of concepts and values runs the risk of displacing "the interpersonal with the technological," to use Plum's (1981, p. 3) phrase. Finally, focusing on a set of action *skills* perpetuates the use of the action model of communication with its focus on only one person in an interaction. Nevertheless, given all these concerns, I have found it helpful to specify particular behavioral skills that *reflect the intent* to be empathic. Ten such behaviors are presented in Table 8-1.

This list of behavioral skills is not exhaustive, nor are the definitions standardized ones. In fact, I refine the list continually (Pickering, 1986; Pickering & VanRheenen, 1984). Furthermore, numerous writers in interpersonal communication, the helping professions, counseling, and parenting have delineated empathic and other helping skills. See, for example, Brammer (1985), Faber and Mazlish (1980), Gordon (1970), Hill (1982), and Marshall, Kurtz, and Associates (1982).

Presenting a construct's opposite is an additional way to learn about it. To this end, Table 8-2 identifies behaviors associated with the intent to listen as a *critic,* with no desire to understand a student's perspective.

Certainly, neither this list of behaviors nor the set of examples is definitive. Listening as a critic, failing to confirm the other, and inducing alienation have all been examined by various scholars. For detailed discussions, Kelly (1982), Gordon (1970), and Laing (1967) are particularly helpful.

Because empathy is a major component of helping relationships, understanding the associated skills as well as their obverse should contribute to enhanced interpersonal communication in the supervisory process. A major caveat needs to be presented, however. I am not suggesting that nonevaluative empathy is always the best way to be with students in the supervisory process. It is but one way. An interesting critique of empathy as a construct can be found in an essay by Arnett and Nakagawa (1983). Further, an alternative to empathy, interpretive or dialogic listening, is discussed by Stewart

Table 8-1. *Behavioral Skills Associated with Empathy*

Behavioral Skills	Explanation
1. Attending, acknowledging	Providing verbal or nonverbal awareness of student (e.g., eye contact)
2. Restating, paraphrasing	Responding to student's basic verbal message
3. Reflecting	Reflecting content, experiences, or feelings that have been heard or perceived through cues
4. Interpreting	Offering a tentative interpretation about student's feelings, desires, or meanings
5. Summarizing, synthesizing	Bringing together student's feelings and experiences; providing a focus
6. Supportive questioning	Probing in a way that requests more information or that attempts to clear up confusions
7. Giving feedback	Sharing perceptions of student's ideas or feelings; disclosing relevant personal information
8. Supporting	Showing warmth and caring in one's own individual way
9. Checking perceptions	Finding out if one's interpretations and perceptions are valid and accurate
10. Being quiet	Giving student time to think as well as to talk

Table 8-2. *Behaviors Associated with Listening as a Critic*

Behavior	Example
1. Denying feelings, perceptions, experiences	"There is no reason to be upset, you're not that bad."
2. Advising, insisting, imposing	"Well, I think you *should* talk to the parents; it will be good for you to do that."
3. Judging negatively, admonishing	"You shouldn't have done it that way."
4. Diagnosing or explaining the other's world to that person	"You only feel that way because you're uptight about your practicum grade."
5. Diverting, changing topic	"Here, look at these reports."
6. Giving false hope or inappropriate reassurance	"I'm sure it'll be all right."
7. Making impersonal, stereotypic statements	"You're just a typical graduate student."
8. Focusing inappropriately on one's self	"Why, that happened to me the other day. You know..."
9. Interrogating	"Why on earth did you say *that* to her?"
10. Trivializing	"Oh, that's a silly thing to worry about."

(1983) and Stewart and Thomas (1986). Additional discussions on empathy can be found in Hill (1982), Pickering and VanRheenen (1984–85), and the references noted earlier.

CONCLUSION

This chapter reflects my personal efforts to make sense out of aspects of the supervisory process and supervisory interactions. As I conclude, I am aware that I hold several basic assumptions or convictions:

1. If interpersonal communication is to be focused on in the preparation of practitioners in Human Communication Disorders, practicum supervisors are the ones most likely to do so.

2. Humanistic-existential thought presents a hopeful view of people and their capability for change. In addition, it provides some direction for working in helping relationships.

3. The field of Interpersonal Communication provides a rich literature for understanding the nature of dyadic communication.

4. The transactional model of communication is the most comprehensive model to date for understanding and analyzing interpersonal communication.

5. Empathic communication is one of the important ways of communicating with student–clinicians.

6. Two new areas that have great potential to inform our understanding of the supervisory process and supervisory interactions are the human sciences and feminist hermeneutics. (See Chapter 5 for a discussion of the human sciences in particular.)

My major conclusion at this point is that making sense out of supervisory endeavors is a never-ending, challenging process. To this end, I find the words of philosopher Charles Virtue (personal communication) meaningful:

> The end of all our seeking
>   the strength of all our knowing
>   the light of all our striving
>   is the seeking
> Itself
> Meanwhile, there is work to do.
> Peace.

REFERENCES

Andrews, J. R. & Andrews, M. A. (1984, November). *A family systems approach to speech–language habilitative services.* Miniseminar presented at the meeting of the American Speech–Language–Hearing Association, San Francisco, CA.

Arnett, R. C. & Nakagawa, E. (1983). The assumptive roots of empathic listening: A critique. *Communication Education, 32,* 368–378.

Bateson, G. (1972). *Steps to an ecology of mind.* New York: Ballantine Books.

Bennis, W. G., Schein, E. R., Steele, F. A. & Berlew, D. E. (1980). Towards better interpersonal relationships. In B. W. Morse & L. A. Phelps (Eds.), *Interpersonal communication: A relational perspective* (pp. 65–80). Minneapolis, MN: Burgess Publishing.

Boone, D. R. & Prescott, T. E. (1972). Content and sequence analysis of speech and hearing therapy. *Asha, 14,* 58–62.

Brammer, L. M. (1985). *The helping relationship* (3rd ed.). Englewood Cliffs, NJ: Prentice-Hall.

Buber, M. (1958). *I and thou* (2nd ed.) (R. G. Smith, Trans.). New York: Charles Scribner's Sons.

Buber, M. (1965). *Between man and man* (R. G. Smith, Trans.). New York: Macmillan.

Buber, M. (1966). *The knowledge of man* (M. Friedman & R. G. Smith, Trans., M. Friedman, Ed.). New York: Harper Torchbooks, Harper & Row.

Buhler, C. (1971). Basic theoretical concepts of humanistic psychology. *American Psychologist, 26,* 378–386.

Campbell, E. (1984). Humanistic psychology: The end of innocence. *Journal of Humanistic Psychology, 24*(2), 6–29.

Caracciolo, G. L., Rigrodsky, S. & Morrison, E. B. (1978a). A Rogerian orientation to the speech–language pathology supervisory relationship. *Asha, 20,* 286–290.

Caracciolo, G. L., Rigrodsky, S. & Morrison, E. B. (1978b). Perceived interpersonal conditions and professional growth of master's level speech–language pathology students during the supervisory process. *Asha, 20,* 467–477.

Collier, H. (1982). *Counseling women: A guide for therapists.* New York: The Free Press. A Division of Macmillian.

Conant, S. & Budoff, M. (1984). Language intervention: Objectivity, engagement, and the clinician's roles. *Journal of Childhood Communication Disorders, 7*(2), 55–64.

Crago, M. (1983, November). *Student supervisor interactional self-exploratory training: A description and model.* Short course presented at the meeting of the American Speech–Language–Hearing Association, Cincinnati, OH.

Egan, G. (1975). *The skilled helper.* Monterey, CA: Brooks/Cole.

Emerick, L. L. & Hood, S. B. (Eds.). (1974). *The client–clinician relationship.* Springfield, IL: Charles C Thomas.

Faber, A. & Mazlish, E. (1980). *How to talk so kids will listen and listen so kids will talk.* New York: Rawson, Wade.

Farmer, S. S. (1986a). Facilitating interpersonal communication competence in supervisory conflict systems. *SUPERvision, 10*(1), 23–26 (Summary).

Farmer, S. S. (1986b). Verbal and nonverbal interpersonal communication pacing: A facilitative program. *SUPERvision, 10*(2), 16–25 (Summary).

Farmer, S. S. (1985–86). Relationship development in supervisory conferences: A tripartite view of the process. *The Clinical Supervisor, 3*(4), 5–21.

Frankl, V. E. (1963). *Man's search for meaning.* New York: Washington Square Press.

Garvin, B. J. & Kennedy, C. W. (1986). Confirmation and disconfirmation in nurse/physician communication. *Journal of Applied Communication Research, 14*(1), 1–19.

Gordon, T. (1970). *Parent effectiveness training.* New York: New American Library.

Greenspan, M. (1983). *A new approach to women and therapy.* New York: McGraw-Hill.

Hagler, P. (1985). Some preliminary effects of communication skills training for speech pathology students at two levels of clinical experience. *SUPERvision, 9*(2), 2–6.

Hill, S. E. (1982). The multistage process of interpersonal empathy. In S. E. Hill, (Ed.), *Improving interpersonal competence: A laboratory approach* (pp. 83–89). Dubuque, IA: Kendall/Hunt.

Hocker, J. L. & Wilmot, W. W. (1985). *Interpersonal conflict* (2nd ed.). Dubuque, IA: Wm. C. Brown.

Hubbell, R. D. (1981). *Children's language disorders.* Englewood Cliffs, NJ: Prentice-Hall.

Ivey, A. E. & Galvin, M. (1983). Skills training: A model for treatment. In E. K. Marshall, P. D. Kurtz & Associates, *Interpersonal helping skills* (pp. 471–481). San Francisco, CA: Jossey-Bass.

Kaplan, N. R. & Dreyer, D. E. (1974). The effect of self-awareness training on student speech pathologist–client relationships. *Journal of Communication Disorders, 7,* 329–342.

Kelly, C. M. (1982). Empathic listening. In J. Stewart (Ed.), *Bridges not walls* (3rd ed.) (pp. 214–218). Reading, MA: Addison-Wesley.

Klevans, D. R. & Volz, H. B. (1978). Interpersonal skill development for speech clinicians. *Journal National Student Speech and Hearing Association, 6,* 63–69.

Klevans, D. R., Volz, H. B., Fiore, M. & Love, C. (1980–81). Parents' and adult clients' preferences for different verbal interaction styles. *SUPERvision, 4*(4), 10–13 (Summary).

Klevans, D. R., Volz, H. B. & Friedman, R. M. (1981). A comparison of experiential and observational approaches for enhancing the interpersonal communication skills of speech–language pathology students. *Journal of Speech and Hearing Disorders, 46,* 208–213.

Kübler-Ross, E. (1969). *On death and dying.* New York: Macmillan.

Laing, R. D. (1967). *The politics of experience.* New York: Pantheon Books, A Division of Random House.

Luterman, D. (1979). *Counseling parents of hearing-impaired children.* Boston, MA: Little, Brown.

McCrea, E. S. (1980). Supervisee ability to self-explore and four facilitative dimensions of supervisor behavior in individual conferences in speech–language pathology (Doctoral dissertation, Indiana University, 1980). *Dissertation Abstracts International, 41*(6), 2134-B. (University Microfilm No. 80-29, 239)

Marshall, E. K., Kurtz, P. D. & Associates. (1982). *Interpersonal helping skills.* San Francisco, CA: Jossey-Bass.

Maslow, A. H. (1966). *The psychology of science: A reconnaissance.* Chicago, IL: Henry Regnery.

Moore, J. C. (1979). Clinical training and the interpersonal relationship. *SUPERvision, 3*(2), 9–12.

Murphy, A. (1982). The clinical process and the speech–language pathologist. In G. H. Shames & E. H. Wiig (Eds.), *Human communication disorders: An introduction* (pp. 453–474). Columbus, OH: Charles E. Merrill.

Oratio, A. R. (1977). *Supervision in speech pathology: A handbook for supervisors and clinicians.* Baltimore, MD: University Park Press.

Oratio, A. R. (1979a). Computer assisted interaction analysis in speech–language pathology and audiology. *Asha, 21,* 179–184.

Oratio, A. R. (1979b). *Pattern recognition: A computer program for interaction analysis of intervention and training processes in speech and hearing.* Baltimore, MD: University Park Press.

Pedersen, P. (1982). Cross-cultural triad model. In E. K. Marshall, P. D. Kurtz & Associates, *Interpersonal helping skills* (pp. 238–284). San Francisco, CA: Jossey-Bass.

Pickering, M. (1977). An examination of concepts operative in the supervisory process and relationship. *Asha, 19,* 607–610.

Pickering, M. (1981). Supervising student teachers: How to provide non-threatening feedback. *Journal of Childhood Communication Disorders, 5*(2), 150–153.

Pickering, M. (1984). Interpersonal communication in speech–language pathology supervisory conferences: A qualitative study. *Journal of Speech and Hearing Disorders, 49,* 189–195.

Pickering, M. (1985). Interpersonal communication constructs and principles: Applications in clinical work. In C. S. Simon (Ed.), *Communication skills and classroom success: Therapy methodologies for language–learning disabled students* (pp. 95–110). San Diego, CA: College-Hill Press.

Pickering, M. (1986). Communication. *Explorations, A Journal of Research at the University of Maine,* III(1), 16–19.

Pickering, M. & McCready, V. (1983). Supervisory journals: An 'inside' look at supervision. *SUPERvision, 7*(1), 5–7 (Summary).

Pickering, M. & VanRheenen, D. D. (1984). Interpersonal communication in clinical and supervisory relationships: Skills, research, theory. *SUPERvision, 8*(2), 2–7 (Summary).

Pickering, M. & VanRheenen, D. D. (1984–85). Supervisory conferences: A place for teaching interpersonal communication concepts, skills. *SUPERvision, 8*(4), 2–11 (Summary).

Pickering, M. & VanRheenen, D. D. (1985, November). *Clinical and supervisory communication processes: A relational systems perspective.* Miniseminar presented at the meeting of the American Speech-Language-Hearing Association, Washington, DC.

Plum, A. (1981). Communication as skill: A critique and alternative proposal. *Journal of Humanistic Psychology, 21*(4), 3–19.

Roberts, J. E. & Smith, K. J. (1982). Supervisor–supervisee role differences and consistency of behavior in supervisory conferences. *Journal of Speech and Hearing Research, 25,* 428–434.

Rogers, C. (1958). The characteristics of a helping relationship. *Personnel and Guidance Journal, 37,* 6–16.

Rosenthal, W. S. (1977, November). *Peer group therapy for beginning clinicians.* Paper presented at the meeting of the American Speech and Hearing Association, Chicago, IL.

Schmitt, J. F. & Gibbs, D. P. (1984–85). Interpersonal skills in clinical supervision: An investigation of efficacy data. *SUPERvision, 8*(4), 12–15 (Summary).

Searle, J. R. (1983). *Intentionality.* Cambridge, England: Cambridge University Press.

Shriberg, L. D., Filley, F. S., Hayes, D. M., Kwiatkowski, J., Schatz, J. A., Simmons, K. M. & Smith, M. E. (1975). The Wisconsin procedure for appraisal of clinical competence (W-PACC): Model and data. *Asha, 17,* 158–165.

Sieburg, E. (1985). *Family communication: An integrated systems approach.* New York: Gardner Press.

Smith, D. R. & Williamson, L. K. (1985). *Interpersonal communication: Roles, rules, strategies, and games* (3rd ed.). Dubuque, IA: Wm. C. Brown.

Smith, K. J. & Anderson, J. L. (1982). Relationship of perceived effectiveness to verbal interaction/content variables in supervisory conferences in speech–language pathology. *Journal of Speech and Hearing Research, 25,* 252–261.

Sorenson, D. (1983, November). *Communicator style characteristics of speech pathology/audiology students.* Paper presented at the meeting of the American-Speech-Language-Hearing Association, Cincinnati, OH.

Stewart, J. (1983). Interpretive listening: An alternative to empathy. *Communication Education, 32,* 379–391.

Stewart J. (Ed.). (1986). *Bridges not walls* (4th ed.). New York: Random House.

Stewart, J. & Thomas, M. (1986). Dialogic listening: Sculpting mutual meanings. In J. Stewart (Ed.), *Bridges not walls* (4th ed.) (pp. 180–196). New York: Random House.

Teilhard de Chardin, P. (1959). *The phenomenon of man.* New York: Harper & Row.

Volz, H. B., Klevans, D. R., Norton, S. J. & Putens, D. L. (1978). Interpersonal communication skills of speech–language pathology undergraduates: The effects of training. *Journal of Speech and Hearing Disorders, 43,* 524–542.

Ward, L. M., Antwine, B. M., Hillard, S. W., Covington, J. R. & Barker, L. (1984, November). *Communicative strategies for improving supervision.* Short course presented at the meeting of the American Speech-Language-Hearing Association, San Francisco, CA.

Ward, L. M. & Webster, E. J. (1965a). The training of clinical personnel: I. Issues in conceptualization. *Asha, 7,* 38–40.

Ward, L. M. & Webster, E. J. (1965b). The training of clinical personnel: II. A concept of clinical preparation. *Asha, 7,* 103–106.

Watzlawick, P. & Weakland, J. H. (1977). *The interactional view.* New York: W. W. Norton.

Wilder, C. (1979). The Palo Alto group: Difficulties and directions of the interactional view for human communication research. *Human Communication Research, 5*(2), 171–186.

Wilmot, W. W. (1979). *Dyadic communication* (2nd ed.). Reading, MA: Addison-Wesley.

Author Index

Subject Index